Parasites, Zoonoses and War

Parasites, Zoonoses and War

A Themed Issue in Honor of Emeritus Professor John M Goldsmid

Editor

Richard S. Bradbury

MDPI • Basel • Beijing • Wuhan • Barcelona • Belgrade • Manchester • Tokyo • Cluj • Tianjin

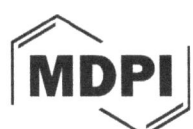

Editor
Richard S. Bradbury
Centers for Disease Control
and Prevention
USA

Editorial Office
MDPI
St. Alban-Anlage 66
4052 Basel, Switzerland

This is a reprint of articles from the Special Issue published online in the open access journal *Tropical Medicine and Infectious Disease* (ISSN 2414-6366) (available at: https://www.mdpi.com/journal/tropicalmed/special_issues/Goldsmid).

For citation purposes, cite each article independently as indicated on the article page online and as indicated below:

LastName, A.A.; LastName, B.B.; LastName, C.C. Article Title. *Journal Name* **Year**, *Article Number*, Page Range.

ISBN 978-3-03936-631-6 (Pbk)
ISBN 978-3-03936-632-3 (PDF)

Cover image courtesy of Ahmed Latif.

© 2020 by the authors. Articles in this book are Open Access and distributed under the Creative Commons Attribution (CC BY) license, which allows users to download, copy and build upon published articles, as long as the author and publisher are properly credited, which ensures maximum dissemination and a wider impact of our publications.

The book as a whole is distributed by MDPI under the terms and conditions of the Creative Commons license CC BY-NC-ND.

Contents

About the Editor vii

Preface to "Parasites, Zoonoses and War" ix

Richard S. Bradbury
Parasites, Zoonoses and War: A Themed Issue in Honor of Emeritus Professor
John M. Goldsmid
Reprinted from: *Trop. Med. Infect. Dis.* **2020**, 5, 103, doi:10.3390/tropicalmed5020103 1

John Goldsmid and Silvana Bettiol
Global Medicine, Parasites, and Tasmania
Reprinted from: *Trop. Med. Infect. Dis.* **2020**, 5, 7, doi:10.3390/tropicalmed5010007 5

Ahmed S. Latif
The Importance of Understanding Social and Cultural Norms in Delivering Quality Health Care—A Personal Experience Commentary
Reprinted from: *Trop. Med. Infect. Dis.* **2020**, 5, 22, doi:10.3390/tropicalmed5010022 15

Richard S. Bradbury
Ternidens deminutus Revisited: A Review of Human Infections with the False Hookworm
Reprinted from: *Trop. Med. Infect. Dis.* **2019**, 4, 106, doi:10.3390/tropicalmed4030106 23

Wayne D. Melrose and Peter A. Leggat
Acute Lymphatic Filariasis Infection in United States Armed Forces Personnel Deployed to the Pacific Area of Operations during World War II Provides Important Lessons for Today
Reprinted from: *Trop. Med. Infect. Dis.* **2020**, 5, 63, doi:10.3390/tropicalmed5020063 35

Gregory M Woods, A. Bruce Lyons and Silvana S Bettiol
A Devil of a Transmissible Cancer
Reprinted from: *Trop. Med. Infect. Dis.* **2020**, 5, 50, doi:10.3390/tropicalmed5020050 41

Ineka Gow, Douglas Millar, John Ellis, John Melki and Damien Stark
Semi-Quantitative, Duplexed qPCR Assay for the Detection of *Leishmania* spp. Using Bisulphite Conversion Technology
Reprinted from: *Trop. Med. Infect. Dis.* **2019**, 4, 135, doi:10.3390/tropicalmed4040135 51

John Frean
Gnathostomiasis Acquired by Visitors to the Okavango Delta, Botswana
Reprinted from: *Trop. Med. Infect. Dis.* **2020**, 5, 39, doi:10.3390/tropicalmed5010039 63

Sarah G. H. Sapp, Monica Kaminski, Marie Abdallah, Henry S. Bishop, Mark Fox, MacKevin Ndubuisi and Richard S. Bradbury
Percutaneous Emergence of *Gnathostoma spinigerum* Following Praziquantel Treatment
Reprinted from: *Trop. Med. Infect. Dis.* **2019**, 4, 145, doi:10.3390/tropicalmed4040145 71

Harsha Sheorey
e-Diagnosis in Medical Parasitology
Reprinted from: *Trop. Med. Infect. Dis.* **2020**, 5, 8, doi:10.3390/tropicalmed5010008 77

About the Editor

Richard S. Bradbury has an extensive background in parasitology, one health, zoonoses, and diagnostics. He has an undergraduate degree majoring in Medical Laboratory Science and has over twelve years of experience working in diagnostic Microbiology and Parasitology laboratories. He completed his PhD at the University of Tasmania (UTAS) in 2010, while working at the Royal Hobart Hospital. After completion of his PhD, he became a Lecturer in Medical Microbiology at UTAS and started capacity building and training in Microbiology and Parasitology diagnostics in Kupang, Indonesia. He also began work on soil-transmitted helminth (STH) infections in the Solomon Islands, including training local laboratory staff in STH screening. He moved to the Keneba field station of the MRC The Gambia in 2012 and managed the laboratory, including training local staff and undertaking parasite surveillance studies. In 2013, he moved to Central Queensland University. Here, he undertook work on surveillance of Strongyloides stercoralis in North Queensland and STH in the Solomon Islands. In 2016, Dr Bradbury was appointed as the Team Lead of the Parasitology Reference Diagnostic Laboratory at the Centers for Disease Control and Prevention (CDC) in the USA. His role was to manage all aspects of the laboratory, including the CDC DPDx parasitology training web site. He continued to teach laboratory diagnostic parasitology in CDC training workshops, lectures, and webinars. Dr Bradbury recently returned to Australia and began a position at Federation University. Here, he is continuing his work on parasite diagnostics, training and capacity building in resource poor nations, and surveillance of STH and other parasitic diseases.

Preface to "Parasites, Zoonoses and War"

It is with the greatest of pleasures that I preface this book dedicated to the life and work of Professor John Marsden Goldsmid. John Goldsmid studied entomology at Rhodes University in South Africa, graduating with an M.Sc. based on finding the host behaviour of tick larvae. While at Rhodes, he met his future wife, Hilary, and after completing his M.Sc. research, he moved to Rhodesia (now Zimbabwe), where Hilary was working as a teacher. For a short while he worked as an entomologist but then moved back into academia, being appointed to a teaching position in the Zoology Department at the University of Rhodesia and Nyasaland. With the formation of the Medical School at what had become the University of Rhodesia (now University of Zimbabwe), John transferred to the Pathology Department, and then to the newly formed Department of Medical Microbiology. John and Hilary were married in Salisbury, and Hilary provided magnificent support and encouragement throughout John's career.

The post at the University also involved running the Parasitology Department of the Harare Hospital Pathology Laboratory, and this allowed John to develop his interest in parasitic diseases and zoonoses based on the many rare and exotic parasitoses that he encountered in the laboratory. He concentrated on the intestinal nematode infections of humans, especially the hookworm disease and ternidensiasis.

John completed his Ph.D. at the University of London, under the inspiring supervision of Professor George Nelson of the London School of Hygiene and Tropical Medicine, and was appointed as Professor and Head of the Department of Medical Microbiology, continuing and extending his research into parasitic and other infections, and their identification, diagnosis, and treatment.

At this point, Professor Goldsmid was commissioned into the army Medical Corps (now the Zimbabwe National Army Medical Corps) and became involved in developing a diagnostic parasitology laboratory for the medical corps. With the extension of the hostilities in the country, and the employment of army and police personnel into the more remote parts of Central Africa, the army was acutely aware of the problem and dangers of infectious and parasitic diseases, and thus, the lab was developed.

In 1977, John emigrated to Australia and became a senior lecturer at the School of Medicine at the University of Tasmania. Here, he taught microbiology and continued his passionate work in parasitology and zoonotic diseases. He became an advocate for parasitology within professional organisations such as the Australian Society for Microbiology and the Australasian College of Tropical Medicine and edited the journals of both societies for an extended period of time. He also was an early promoter of the field of travel medicine, establishing an early Tropical and Travel Medicine Elective unit at the University of Tasmania.

Professor Goldsmid's impact as a diagnostician, researcher, teacher, and mentor has influenced many in the field of parasitic and zoonotic disease, and it is fitting that this Special Edition of Tropical Medicine and Infectious Diseases is devoted to honouring his outstanding work in these fields, both within Australia and internationally.

Emeritus Professor Goldsmid continued to teach at the University of Tasmania until two years ago. He continues to live in Tasmania with Hilary, where he is now retired.

Richard S. Bradbury
Editor

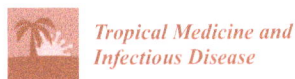

Editorial

Parasites, Zoonoses and War: A Themed Issue in Honor of Emeritus Professor John M. Goldsmid

Richard S. Bradbury

School of Health and Life Sciences, Federation University, Berwick 3806, VIC, Australia; r.bradbury@federation.edu.au; Tel.: +61-3-5327-6584

Received: 16 June 2020; Accepted: 18 June 2020; Published: 21 June 2020

This Special Issue of *Tropical Medicine and Infectious Disease* is dedicated to the life and work of Emeritus Professor John Marsden Goldsmid. Herein, Prof. Goldsmid's colleagues have contributed papers celebrating his academic contribution to the field of parasitology and zoonosis. Prof. Goldsmid's outstanding contributions to medical parasitology, the Australasian College of Tropical Medicine and other learned societies are well known in Australia and elsewhere. He is held in justifiable high esteem. Further to this, Prof. Goldsmid was a gifted teacher and enthusiastic mentor to all those who he touched in his decades working at the University of Tasmania. Prof. Goldsmid's career has included work in the field of parasitology to benefit human and animal health, in peacetime and in war, in both Africa and Australia.

This Special Issue contains a total of nine original, peer-reviewed papers, many of them published by Prof. Goldsmid's former colleagues and co-researchers. Included is a paper co-authored by Prof. Goldsmid himself with Dr. Silvana Bettiol, reflecting on the changes in global medicine, parasites, and Tasmania over the 50 years spanning his career [1]. Further reflection on a lifetime of practice is provided by Prof. Ahmed Latif, a former colleague of Prof. Goldsmid, who summarizes his experience on the importance of cultural understanding in the delivery of healthcare while working as a medical practitioner in Africa and remote Australian Aboriginal communities [2].

Prof Goldsmid focused on human and wildlife diseases in Tasmania in the latter years of his career, often in conjunction with Dr. Silvana Bettiol. In keeping with this, Dr. Bettiol, Dr. Bruce Lyons and Emeritus Prof. Greg Woods from the University of Tasmania have contributed a thought-provoking review of Tasmanian devil facial tumour disease (DFTD). This review takes the novel and engaging approach of comparing aspects of the transmissibility and life cycle of DFTD with that of parasitic organisms and, in so doing, provides an easily accessible analogy for the understanding of the epidemiology of this disease of an iconic Tasmanian marsupial [3].

Reflecting the major focus and impact of Prof. Goldsmid's life and work, the majority of the papers in this issue focus on parasitic diseases. A review of human infections with the false hookworm, *Ternidens deminutus*, described work on the epidemiology, clinical manifestations, pathology, diagnosis and treatment of this neglected helminthic disease, much of it summarizing seminal work performed by Prof. Goldsmid himself in Zimbabwe during the 1960's and 1970's [4].

Prof. Goldsmid promoted the field of travel medicine in its infancy. This theme and that of African parasitic zoonoses are further explored in a case series by Prof. John Frean of the South African National Institute for Communicable Diseases and the University of the Witwatersrand, describing five human cases of gnathostomiasis acquired by travelers to Botswana [5]. Travel-acquired gnathostomiasis is further explored in a report describing another case in a traveler, by Dr. Sarah Sapp and colleagues from the Centers for Disease Control and Prevention and the New York City Health and Hospitals Corporation. This report describes the discovery of a sub-adult *Gnathostoma spinigerum*, which emerged from the skin of a traveler from Bangladesh in temporal association with the patient receiving praziquantel treatment for suspected schistosomiasis [6].

Chronic parasitic infections in military veterans was another area of research to which Prof. Goldsmid provided several important contributions. This theme is admirably addressed by Assoc. Prof. Wayne Melrose and Prof. Peter Leggat, who describe and discuss the modern implications of the outbreak of lymphatic filariasis (LF) in United States armed forces deployed to the Pacific Islands during World War 2. Not only do these authors provide a comprehensive summary of this outbreak and its long term impact on those affected veterans, they also use it as an example of why care must be taken to avoid resurgences of LF in the many Pacific islands where elimination has recently been achieved [7].

The diagnosis of parasitic diseases was a major focus of Prof. Goldsmid's research and this theme is admirably addressed in the work by Dr. Inega Gow, supervised by Dr. Damien Stark, describing the development and validation of a novel real-time PCR assay for the detection, identification and semi-quantitation of *Leishmania* spp. causing cutaneous leishmaniasis [8]. Recognizing Prof. Goldsmid's prodigious knowledge and capability in the diagnosis of difficult and exotic parasitic zoonoses, Dr. Harsha Sheorey contributes an engaging and informative summary of the use of e-diagnosis for the identification of diagnostically challenging parasitic infections and its application to modern cases in medical parasitology [9].

This collection of papers are a testament to the many diverse topics and special areas that Prof. Goldsmid worked on in his distinguished career. The wide range of topics, such as medical parasitology, marsupial diseases in Tasmania, infections in travelers and military veterans, cultural aspects of medical practice, rare zoonotic infections in both Africa and Australia, and the diagnosis of parasitic diseases, reflect the diversity and depth of Prof. Goldsmid's work. Prof. Goldsmid's contributions define him as a great parasitologist, a great Tasmanian, and a great Australian, whose career and life's work has had a substantial impact in the field of parasitology and zoonoses in Australia and Africa. We hope that his prodigious work, deep care for the health and lives of others, and inspiration of younger parasitologists, has been appropriately recognized and reflected in a small part by the high quality and wide variety of papers published in this special edition in his honor.

Funding: This work received no external funding.

Conflicts of Interest: The author declares no conflict of interest.

References

1. Goldsmid, J.; Bettiol, S. Global medicine, parasites, and Tasmania. *Trop. Med. Infect. Dis.* **2020**, *5*, 7. [CrossRef] [PubMed]
2. Latif, A.S. The importance of understanding social and cultural norms in delivering quality health care—A personal experience commentary. *Trop. Med. Infect. Dis.* **2020**, *5*, 22. [CrossRef] [PubMed]
3. Woods, G.M.; Lyons, A.B.; Bettiol, S.S. A devil of a transmissible cancer. *Trop. Med. Infect. Dis.* **2020**, *5*, 50. [CrossRef] [PubMed]
4. Bradbury, R.S. *Ternidens deminutus* revisited: A review of human infections with the false hookworm. *Trop. Med. Infect. Dis.* **2019**, *4*, 106. [CrossRef] [PubMed]
5. Frean, J. Gnathostomiasis acquired by visitors to the Okavango delta, Botswana. *Trop. Med. Infect. Dis.* **2020**, *5*, 39. [CrossRef] [PubMed]
6. Sapp, S.G.; Kaminski, M.; Abdallah, M.; Bishop, H.S.; Fox, M.; Ndubuisi, M.; Bradbury, R.S. Percutaneous emergence of *Gnathostoma spinigerum* following praziquantel treatment. *Trop. Med. Infect. Dis.* **2019**, *4*, 145. [CrossRef] [PubMed]
7. Melrose, W.D.; Leggat, P.A. Acute Lymphatic filariasis infection in United States armed forces personnel deployed to the Pacific area of operations during World War II provides important lessons for today. *Trop. Med. Infect. Dis.* **2020**, *5*, 63. [CrossRef] [PubMed]

8. Gow, I.; Millar, D.; Ellis, J.; Melki, J.; Stark, D. Semi-quantitative, duplexed qPCR assay for the detection of *Leishmania* spp. using bisulphite conversion technology. *Trop. Med. Infect. Dis.* **2019**, *4*, 135. [CrossRef] [PubMed]
9. Sheorey, H. E-diagnosis in medical parasitology. *Trop. Med. Infect. Dis.* **2020**, *5*, 8. [CrossRef] [PubMed]

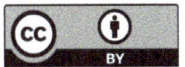

© 2020 by the author. Licensee MDPI, Basel, Switzerland. This article is an open access article distributed under the terms and conditions of the Creative Commons Attribution (CC BY) license (http://creativecommons.org/licenses/by/4.0/).

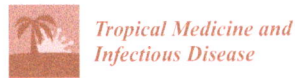

Communication

Global Medicine, Parasites, and Tasmania

John Goldsmid and Silvana Bettiol *

School of Medicine, College of Health and Medicine, University of Tasmania, 17 Liverpool Street, Hobart Tasmania 7000, Australia; j.m.goldsmid@utas.edu.au
* Correspondence: s.bettiol@utas.edu.au; Tel.: +61-3-6226-4826

Received: 6 November 2019; Accepted: 30 December 2019; Published: 1 January 2020

Abstract: Until the 1970s, infectious disease training in most medical schools was limited to those diseases common in the area of instruction. Those wishing to explore a more globalised curriculum were encouraged to undertake specialist postgraduate training at schools or institutes of tropical medicine. However, the increase in global trade and travel from the 1970s onward led to dramatic changes in the likelihood of returning travellers and new immigrants presenting with tropical infections in temperate regions. Furthermore, population growth and the changing relationships between animals, the environment, and man in agriculture accentuated the importance of a wider understanding of emerging infectious diseases, zoonotic diseases and parasitic infections. These epidemiological facts were not adequately reflected in the medical literature or medical curriculum at the time. The orientation on tropical infections needed specialised attention, including instruction on diagnosis and treatment of such infections. We describe key global health events and how the changing field of global medicine, from the 1970s to early 2000, impacted on medical education and research. We describe the impact of global health changes in the Tasmanian context, a temperate island state of Australia. We retrospectively analysed data of patients diagnosed with parasites and present a list of endemic and non-endemic parasites reported during this period. Finally, we reflect on the new approaches to the changing needs of global health and challenges that medical programmes, learners and educators face today.

Keywords: parasitology; zoonoses; tropical medicine; travel medicine; global medicine; Tasmania

1. Introduction

In 1964 and based on concerns regarding tropical disease in temperate climates, Dr. Kevin Cahill published a series of articles in The New York State Journal of Medicine. He foresaw that inexpensive boat travel and the shortening transit times by air travel posed a potential infection hazard [1]. By 1974, Woodruff in the preface to his book stated that "Medicine in the tropics is of great importance to all practitioners be they working in temperate or tropical regions" [2]. He had already noted that through travel "even in temperate regions, a significant proportion of the community has now been exposed to disease in tropical and subtropical regions" [2]. What he said then is even more important now with more global connections involving travel and trade, changes in climate, and the environment and human spread into previously uninhabited regions. These factors have led to the possibility of diseases with short incubation periods being brought to countries where they have not been seen before or have been exceedingly rare. Diseases with long and silent incubation periods present the most difficult diagnostic and public health problems. This, has led to growing clinical needs and development of medical practitioners, public health and health professionals with an understanding of these diseases, working at the local, regional, national, and global level. For those teaching and developing medical curricula these diseases present many challenges and have become more complex due to the changing focus of healthcare systems, globalisation, cultural and societal factors, and technology. Despite international communications on medical education to address these needs, medical practice remains distinctly different among countries [3].

2. Time Line of Selected Global Health Events

Why were the 1970s significant for changes in global medicine? The 1970s was a period when the post-World War II economic expansion and economic boom was drawing to an end and the 1973–1975 recession loomed [4,5]. The economic crisis also affected the approach to the control of disease and much of the work in the field reflected the long-term instability and economic difficulty. The range of effective drugs used for human and animal treatment expanded rapidly. However, the treatment was not always in parallel with investigations of how these new drugs should be used to the best effect. Transport of livestock from country to country without an understanding of disease risks and intensive methods of animal management posed hazards to humans [2,6]. Preparing for reduced funding for medical and veterinary services to make further gains in health and wellbeing of humans and animals was not expected. Promoting efficient use of resources was common and a need for evaluation was obvious.

The growing efficiency and reach of modern transport networks led to an emergence of new strains of familiar diseases, as well as completely new diseases. A consequence was the pressure on how to tackle them. It became apparent that there was strong correlation between antibiotic use in the treatment of humans and animals and antibiotic resistance in Gram-negative pathogens. The most prevalent Gram-negative pathogens at this time were *Escherichia coli*, *Salmonella enterica*, and *Klebsiella pneumoniae* [7]. Since then there has been an alarming increase in 'superbugs' and a decline in the development of new antibiotics to cope with the changing situation. Williamson et al. [8] recently highlighted the danger of drug resistance in *Candida auris*, carbapenemase-producing enterobacteriaceae, Methicillin-resistant *Staphylococcus aureus* (MRSA) and drug-resistant strains of typhoid and gonorrhoea. Infectious disease specialists note that the world has reached a crisis in the treatment of bacterial infections [9,10].

Between 1965 and 1970, the growth rate of the world's population reached its peak, increasing by 2.1% per year on average [11]. There was a growing concern of the impact of this population growth on the interaction of humans and the environment and how this would affect tropical diseases. A combination of increased economic activity, human migration, tourism, and encroachment on new environmental niches contributed to the emergence of many zoonotic diseases. The first cases of naturally acquired *Plasmodium knowlesi* infection [12], the Marburg, Ebola, and Lassa fever viruses [13], and reports of Lyme disease [14] occurred during this period. The earliest reports of a syndrome later identified as HIV/AIDS appeared in the closing year of the 1970s [14].

The 1970s saw the rise of preventive medicine and the self-care movements [15]. In the early part of June 1972, the United Nations Conference on the Human Environment in Stockholm considered the need for "a common outlook and for common principles to inspire and guide the peoples of the world in the preservation and enhancement of the human environment" [16]. Following the Stockholm Declaration, global awareness of environmental issues increased dramatically. In 1992, the second United Nations Conference on Environment and Development (UNCED) in Rio de Janeiro represented a major milestone in the evolution of international environmental law [17]. Today, the Sustainable Goals (SDGs) of the United Nations and the Agenda 2030 reflect the spirit of these principles.

The 1970s initiated great strides in global disease control. A successful example was the Onchocerciasis Control programme, which commenced in 1974 [18]. The serious health and socioeconomic repercussions of onchocerciasis and indications of possible control was a catalyst for a convening of a joint USAID/OCCGE/WHO technical meeting [18,19]. The participants included experts in a range of fields including public health, parasitology, epidemiology, entomology, ophthalmology, economics, sociology, and medical geography [18]. The programme brought relief to many communities and with great effort was sustained and continues today, despite difficult circumstances. This programme has become an example of effective public health management and one of the largest intercountry undertakings implemented by the World Health Organization (WHO) [19,20].

The decade of the 1970s closed with the successful eradication of smallpox after a 14-year intensive programme [21] and the beginning of new global control programmes. There were specific efforts to increase efficiency and productivity of healthcare systems during the 1980s, including improvement in maternal and child health and a focus on HIV/AIDS, tuberculosis, and malaria in developing countries. In 1986, the Global Programme on AIDS (GPA) was launched by the World Health Organization [22] followed by the Global Polio Eradication Initiative (GPEI) in 1988, which was led jointly by national governments, the WHO, Rotary International, the US Centers for Disease Control and Prevention (CDC), and UNICEF [22,23].

In 1992, the CDC launched the international campaign to eradicate Guinea worm disease and eliminate dracunculiasis [24]. The 1990s welcomed the evolution of large data-driven research and collaboration with the World Bank commissioned to publish the Global Burden of Disease study. Today this collaboration has over 1800 researchers and contributors from 127 countries [25]. Another significant global achievement at this time was the Global Initiative for Traditional Systems of Health created by the Pan American Health Organisation [26]. Today WHO continues to develop proactive policies and action plans to strengthen the role of traditional and complementary medicine (T&CM) in responding to health needs of populations. Unfortunately, it remains an ongoing challenge for countries trying to implement regulations and national laws for their use [26].

The next factor which influenced human health over these years, and more evident today, was climate change. Changing climate, spread of warmer conditions, and changing rainfall can increase the occurrence of tropical diseases such as malaria, dengue and schistosomiasis and potentially soil transmitted helminthiases by extending their distribution [27]. Changing climate, including pollution, exacerbates public health issues and economic stagnation due to parasitic diseases and these complexities have been highlighted by numerous authors [28–31]. Thus, Han et al. [32] stated that "Health organisations are growing more concerned that climate change will cause zoonotic diseases to become more prolific and widespread" and challenges are more difficult in predicting outbreaks caused by either novel pathogens or known pathogens in novel places.

The continued pressure of economic development has increased the opportunity for pathogens (many previously unknown) with zoonotic potential to cross the species line. The world's population has continued to grow from 3.7 billion in the 1970s to 7.7 billion in 2019 [33] and is projected to increase to 9.7 billion by 2050. Health professionals need to be aware of growth rates and mobility patterns across their regions [34]. Goldsmid [35] noted "that never before in the history of the human race, have so many people been able to travel so far so quickly and so cheaply"—and this is even truer today!

A review of the literature estimates the number of people that acquire an infectious disease during or as a result of travel ranges from 6% to 87% [36]. These figures may change as current projections suggest the annual number of international travellers will reach 1.8 billion by 2030 [36]. International tourism in Australia for example has grown significantly in the past two decades. The number of short-term overseas visitor arrivals rose from 2.5 million in 1992 to 9.3 million in 2018–2019, the highest year on record [37]. Outbound international trips have nearly doubled in the past decade. The scale and speed of contemporary international travel means an increasing possibility of travellers being exposed to unfamiliar infections.

Accurate data of the proportion of people who acquire an illness overseas are difficult to calculate as exposure is dependent on the destination, baseline medical history, and also planned activities [38]. In recent years research in travel medicine has grown. There are tropical medicine surveillance networks, such as the GeoSentinel surveillance network composed of International Society of Travel Medicine (ISTM) travel and tropical medicine clinics that collect post-travel illness surveillance data [39,40], but there are limitations. Therefore, physicians need to be familiar with destination-specific disease risks, travel and routine vaccines, and chemoprophylaxis regimens. Reviews of current evidence in the discipline are readily available [41].

A major area of medical relevance in the fields of tropical travel, migrant and refugee medicine is parasitic infections. The estimates of the prevalence and incidence of neglected tropical diseases and malaria from the Global Burden of Disease Study 2017 [42] are thought provoking. While some parasitic diseases such as falciparum malaria and human African trypanosomiasis (East African variety) cause acute infections with a high mortality, most parasitic infections are chronic infections. An example is cysticercosis [43–45] which is increasingly recorded in non-endemic regions around the world [43].

3. Historical Overview of Tasmania and Parasites of Medical Importance

Historically, nearly all of the infectious diseases seen in Australia, and especially Tasmania, have been imported since European/Asian settlement of the continent [46] and many of the commoner infections then became endemic as the population grew. Tasmania has a long history associated with imported infections, starting with the first settlement by Europeans (especially the convicts) and continuing from there. Tasmania provides a strong case against a parochial approach to medicine – especially in the changing world today. It is a good model for study in relation to imported infections and the relevance of travel in this regard. The reasons are:

(1) Tasmania is a small relatively isolated island, protected by surrounding water.
(2) Tasmania has a temperate climate with a high standard of living and with good health services.
(3) Tasmania has a small resident population and consequently has fewer overseas travellers or returning travellers.
(4) Tasmania has few direct overseas connections and fewer overseas visitors than the more populous and easily accessible mainland states of Australia.

The question thus arises—How big a range of endemic and 'exotic' imported infections has been diagnosed in humans in Tasmania over recent years? A retrospective analysis of recorded cases was completed and is reported below. Helminth infections are summarised in Table 1 and other key parasites diagnosed in Tasmania in Table 2.

Table 1. Helminth infections diagnosed in Tasmania:

Trematodes:	Cestodes:	Nematodes:
Echinostoma sp. **	*Echinococcus granulosis* ***	*Ancylostoma duodenale* **
Fasciola hepatica **	*Hymenolepis nana* ***	*Ascaris lumbricoides* ***
Opisthorchis viverrni **	*Taenia saginata* **	*Ascaris suum* *
Schistosoma haematobium **	*Taenia solium* (cysticercosis) **	Cutaneous larva migrans **
Schistosoma mansoni **		*Enterobius vermicularis* *
		Eucoleus aerophilus (*Capilalria aerophila*) *
		Haycocknema perplexum **
		Loa loa **
		Necator americanus **
		Strongyloides stercoralis **
		Toxocara spp. *
		Trichinella pseudospiralis *
		Trichuris trichiura ***
		Trichostrongylus spp. **
		Wuchereria bancrofti lymphatic filariasis and tropical pulmonary eosinophilia **

Key to coding: Endemic cases *, Imported cases **, Endemic and imported cases ***.

In the mid-20th Century, Tasmania experienced one of the highest rates of human hydatid disease in the world [47,48]. *Echinococcus granulosus*, which causes cystic echinococcosis is the only member of the genus *Echinococcus* to be found in Australia. It was introduced during the early period of European settlement and described in domestic animals before 1840 [49]. In the early 1960s, the state government commenced a hydatid control programme across Tasmania aimed at stopping transmission of hydatid disease to humans. By 1996, Tasmania was declared provisionally free of hydatids in dogs and livestock [50].

Table 2. Protozoa and Arthropoda diagnosed in Tasmania.

Protozoa	Arthropoda—Insecta:	Arthropoda—Acarina
Chilomastix mesnili ***	*Cordylobia anthropophaga* **	*Sarcoptes scabiei* *
Cryptosporidium spp. *	*Dermatobia hominis* **	Ixodid ticks *
Cyclospora cayetanensis **	*Tunga penetrans* **	
Dientamoeba fragilis ***	*Pediculus humanus capitis* *	
Endolimax nana ***	*Pediculus humanus corporis* *	
Entamoeba histolytica **		
Entamoeba dispar **		
Entamoeba polecki **		
Entamoeba gingivalis *		
Enteromonas hominis **		
Giardia intestinalis ***		
Leishmania tropica **		
Leishmania braziliensis **		
Pentatrichomonas hominis **		
Plasmodium falciparum **		
Plasmodium malariae **		
Plasmodium ovale **		
Plasmodium vivax **		
Toxoplasma gondii *		
Trichomonas vaginalis *		
Trypanosoma cruzi **		
Acanthocephala; *Moniliformis moniliformis* **		**

Key to coding: Endemic cases *, Imported cases **, Endemic and imported cases ***.

Of the helminth cases, the Tasmanian cases of *Trichinella pseudospiralis* and *Haycocknema perplexum* are the most intriguing as they were the first human cases of these worms ever reported [51–53]. It was first described from a patient in Tasmania by Spratt et al. [54]. Subsequent cases diagnosed had all lived in or visited Tasmania. Many had histories of contact with native animals or eating bush meat and it was thought that the infection was an endemic zoonosis from Tasmania [55,56]. A subsequent case from tropical North Queensland had no contact with Tasmania and a re-evaluation of all the recorded cases showed that they all had contact with the tropical north of Australia. The result that the condition was considered to be endemic there and being redescribed the disease as "tropical parasitic myositis" [57]. However, the most recently reported case from Tasmania had no travel history, except to Melbourne in southern Victoria [56], confirming that *H. perplexum* is indeed endemic to Tasmania. The natural reservoir of *H. perplexum* has not been found to date and the mode of transmission to humans is also unknown. Human *T. pseudospiralis* has subsequently been described from humans in France and Thailand but the enigma of *H. perplexum* continues.

Vaccine development and application to control zoonotic diseases in food animals, companion animals, and wildlife have made a significant impact in reducing the incidence of zoonotic diseases in people [58]. At the same time, biosecurity in Australia has played a critical role in maintaining its reputation as a country free of severe pests and diseases. The Commonwealth Quarantine Service started operations in 1908 and today Biosecurity Australia monitors plant and animal health across Australia. While most infections in Australia have been controlled it has led to over-confidence regarding their importance (or even existence) today. Unfortunately, while ubiquitous protozoan species have been reported in wildlife across Australia [51–61] the life cycles, ecology, and general biology of most parasites of wildlife in Australia are poorly understood. Much of the work to date has been opportunistic with unreliable funding opportunities, but with modern methods and 'omic' technology [62] offering an avenue for major advances in the field, there is potential for renewed support and interest.

An analysis of imported malaria in Tasmania (Table 2) was initially reported over a 5-year period from 1987 to 1992 and subsequently extended to cover 1987–1994 [63]. During this period,

80 cases of malaria were diagnosed covering three species: *Plasmodium vivax* (81.2%) followed by *Plasmodium falciparum* (16.2%), and *Plasmodium malariae* (2.6%). Cases came from Asia, Southeast Asia, Africa, Papua New Guinea (PNG), Vanuatu, the Solomons, and one case acquired in Thursday Island (administratively a part of Australia and an area considered free from malaria due to control measures). The cases were diagnosed from across the State, including two from Antarctica—a region administered from Tasmania (Goldsmid, pers. Comm. 2019). These cases continued to influence curriculum development in tropical and travel disease in the undergraduate medical school. Expanding medical training in tropical disease for Tasmanian medical practitioners was highlighted by one of these malaria cases when originally misdiagnosed (as influenza). The general practitioner (GP) involved explained the patient presented during an influenza epidemic in his area and, as he ruefully admitted, he did not ask the patient about any travel history. Luckily it was a case of benign tertian malaria (*Plasmodium vivax*)—the error could have been tragic if it had been a case of *P. falciparum* malaria

New treatments are, however, being developed, albeit rather slowly and an example of this is the treatment of *Plasmodium vivax* relapses with tafenoquine (kozenis) and artesunate for severe falciparum malaria [64]. The recent and rapid clinical development of vaccines is making considerable impact world-wide. The vaccine against *Plasmodium falciparum*, RTS,S/AS01 (RTS,S) is a promising vaccine candidate for malaria currently part of a landmark pilot program in three African countries, and is available to children up to 2 years of age [65]. Another recent example is the vesicular stomatitis virus-based Ebola virus vaccine (VSV-EBOV) currently in a clinical trial [66]. It is viewed as a potential tool for both current and future Ebola outbreaks.

Infectious diseases and pandemic preparedness remain a priority on the world agenda, despite the shift in focus to non-communicable diseases. The Sustainable Development Goals (SDGs) provide a framework for a holistic answer to the ensuing challenges and respond to these complex interactions but collaboration between research disciplines is essential. A recent paper by committee members of the World Heath Summit supports the view that leading institutions and organisations are responsible to promote transdisciplinary, cross-sectoral, science-based and concerted efforts for more efficient and equitable ways to advance health on a global scale [67].

4. Conclusions

Changing attitudes over the course of several decades mean medicine has slowly been considered in global terms rather than discrete specialties. The changing patterns in disease suggest a need for new conceptual models in medical training and medical education. There have been many attempts to frame the impact of globalisation on health [68] based on international health, public health, and tropical medicine [68–70]. During the period of our work in medical curriculum development and medical microbiology teaching the commoner categories included: tropical medicine, travel medicine, migrant medicine, and traditional and complementary medicine. All of these specialties, to varying degrees, can be encompassed under the broad title of 'Global Medicine'. This has coincided with attempts to integrate modern science into the medical curricula and equip health professionals to meet the future health needs of populations.

The One Health concept recognises the health connections between humans, animals, and their shared environments [71]. Its approach has been endorsed by a number of medical and public health organisations and medical schools around the world [71]. The concept of planetary health, which became part of the fabric of integrative medicine in the 1990s, has since become a concept that has penetrated mainstream academic and medical discourse. In fact, it provides a new multidisciplinary approach to understanding the interconnections between environmental and human health. It is often viewed as a response to existing fields of public health, environmental health, Ecohealth, One Health, and international health [72].

The impressive range of infections currently seen and potentially emergent emphasises what Bradley [73] warned the medical profession over 30 years ago, that a holistic view is one all specialties must embrace. Our work in medical education and our past experiences are still valid today. Tropical diseases are not confined to the tropics. They are being increasingly encountered in non-tropical areas and thus must be considered a global problem.

Author Contributions: J.G. and S.B. both participated substantially in the writing and editing of this manuscript. All authors have read and agreed to the published version of the manuscript.

Funding: This research received no external funding.

Acknowledgments: We thank Richard Bradbury and ACTM for the invitation and opportunity to contribute to this special issue. Thanks to Gregory Woods and Associate Bruce Lyons for reviewing this work.

Conflicts of Interest: The authors declare no conflicts of interest.

References

1. Cahill, K.M. Tropical Diseases in Temperate Climates. Lippincott: Philadelphia, PA, USA; Montreal, QC, Canada, 1964; pp. 1–216.
2. Woodruff, A.W. *Medicine in the Tropics*; Churchill Livingstone: Edinburgh/London, UK, 1974; ISBN 0443009562.
3. O'Brien, B.C.; Forrest, K.; Wijnen-Meijer, M.; ten Cate, O. A Global View of Structures and Trends in Medical Education. In *Understanding Medical Education: Evidence, Theory, and Practice*, 3rd ed.; Swanwick, T., Forrest, K., O'Brien, B.C., Eds.; Wiley-Blackwell: Hoboken, NJ, USA, 2018; pp. 7–22. Available online: https://doi.org/10.1002/9781119373780 (accessed on 27 November 2019).
4. Zarnowitz, V.; Moore, G.H. The recession and recovery of 1973–1976. In *Explorations in Economic Research*; NBER: Cambridge, MA, USA, 1977; Volume 4, pp. 1–87. Available online: https://apps.who.int/gb/ebwha/pdf_files/EB144/B144_22-en.pdf (accessed on 2 October 2019).
5. Marglin, S.A.; Schor, J.B. *The Golden Age of Capitalism: Reinterpreting the Postwar Experience*; Oxford University Press: Oxford, UK, 1991; ISBN 9780198287414.
6. Gubler, D.J. Vector-borne diseases. *Rev. Sci. Tech.* **2009**, *28*, 583–588. [CrossRef]
7. Davies, J.; Davies, D. Origins and evolution of antibiotic resistance. *Microbiol. Mol. Biol. Rev.* **2010**, *74*, 417–433. [CrossRef] [PubMed]
8. Williamson, D.A.; Howden, B.P.; Paterson, D.L. The risk of resistance: What are the major antimicrobial resistance threats facing Australia? *Med. J. Aust.* **2019**, *211*, 103–105. [CrossRef]
9. Hall, W. *Superbugs: An Arms Race Against Bacteria*; Harvard University Press: Cambridge, MA, USA, 2018; pp. 1–256. ISBN 9780674975989.
10. McCarthy, M. *Superbugs: The Race to Stop an Epidemic*; Penguin Random House Audio: New York, NY, USA, 2019; p. 304. ISBN 978-0735217508.
11. Roser, M.; Ritchie, H.; Ortiz-Ospina, E. World Population Growth. Available online: https://ourworldindata.org/world-population-growth (accessed on 27 November 2019).
12. Singh, B.; Daneshvar, C. Human infections and detection of *Plasmodium knowlesi*. *Clin. Microbiol. Rev.* **2013**, *26*, 165–184. [CrossRef]
13. Seah, S.K. Lassa, Marburg and Ebola: Newly described African fevers. *Can. Med. Assoc. J.* **1978**, *118*, 347–348.
14. Ferguson, R. Emerging infectious diseases–1970s. *J. Community Hosp. Intern. Med. Perspect.* **2016**, *6*, 32662. [CrossRef]
15. Prescott, S.L.; Logan, A.C.; Katz, D.L. Preventive Medicine for Person, Place, and Planet: Revisiting the Concept of High-Level Wellness in the Planetary Health Paradigm. *Int. J. Environ. Res. Public Health* **2019**, *16*, 238. [CrossRef] [PubMed]
16. UN General Assembly. In Proceedings of the United Nations Conference on the Human Environment, Stockholm, Sweden, 15 December 1972; A/RES/2994. Available online: https://www.refworld.org/docid/3b00f1c840.html (accessed on 12 November 2019).
17. United Nations. Transforming Our World: The 2030 Agenda for Sustainable Development. *General Assembly 70 Session.* 2015. Available online: https://www.unfpa.org/sites/default/files/resource-pdf/Resolution_A_RES_70_1_EN.pdf (accessed on 10 August 2019).
18. World Health Organization. *Onchocerciasis Control in the Volta River Basin Area: Report of the Mission for Preparatory Assistance to the Governments of Dahomey, Ghana, Ivory Coast, Mali, Niger, Togo and Upper Volta*; (No. OCP/73.1); WHO: Geneva, Switzerland, 1973; Available online: https://apps.who.int/iris/handle/10665/326129 (accessed on 10 August 2019).

19. Samba, E.M.; World Health Organization. *The Onchocerciasis Control Programme in West Africa: An Example of Effective Public Health Management/Ebrahim M. Samba*; WHO: Geneva, Switzerland, 1994; Available online: https://apps.who.int/iris/handle/10665/39261 (accessed on 10 August 2019).
20. Thylefors, B. Onchocerciasis: Impact of interventions. *Community Eye Health* **2001**, *14*, 17–19.
21. World Health Organization. The Smallpox Eradication Programme—SEP (1966–1980). 2010. Available online: https://www.who.int/features/2010/smallpox/en/ (accessed on 31 October 2019).
22. Lisk, F. The rise and fall of the WHO's Global Program on AIDS (GPA). In *Global Institutions and the HIV/AIDS Epidemic: Responding to an International Crisis*; Routledge: London, UK; New York, NY, USA, 2009; pp. 15–27.
23. Henderson, R.H. The World Health Organization's Plan of Action for Global Eradication of Poliomyelitis by the Year 2000. *Ann. N. Y. Acad. Sci.* **1989**, *569*, 69–85. [CrossRef]
24. Centers for Disease Control and Prevention. Parasites—Guinea Worm—Eradication Program. 2019. Available online: https://www.cdc.gov/parasites/guineaworm/gwep.html (accessed on 31 October 2019).
25. Das, P. The story of GBD 2010: A "super human" effort. *Lancet* **2012**, *380*, 2067–2070. [CrossRef]
26. World Health Organization. *WHO Global Report on Traditional and Complementary Medicine 2019*; World Health Organization: Geneva, Switzerland, 2019; Available online: https://apps.who.int/iris/handle/10665/312342 (accessed on 10 December 2019).
27. Weaver, H.J.; Hawdon, J.M.; Hoberg, E.P. Soil-transmitted helminthiases: Implications of climate change and human behavior. *Trends Parasitol.* **2010**, *26*, 574–581. [CrossRef] [PubMed]
28. Andreae, M.O.; Rosenfeld, D.; Artaxo, P.; Costa, A.A.; Frank, G.P.; Longo, K.M.; Silva-Dias, M.A. Smoking rain clouds over the Amazon. *Science* **2004**, *303*, 1309–1311. [CrossRef] [PubMed]
29. Patz, J.A.; Olson, S.H. Climate change and health: Global to local influences on disease risk. *Ann. Trop. Med. Parasitol.* **2006**, *100*, 535–539. [CrossRef] [PubMed]
30. Patz, J.A.; Gibbs, H.K.; Foley, J.A.; Rogers, J.V.; Smith, K.R. Climate change and global health: Quantifying a growing ethical crisis. *EcoHealth* **2007**, *4*, 397–405. [CrossRef]
31. Short, E.E.; Caminade, C.; Thomas, B.N. Climate change contribution to the emergence or re-emergence of parasitic diseases. *Infect. Dis. (Auckl.)* **2017**, *10*, 1–7. [CrossRef]
32. Han, B.A.; Kramer, A.M.; Drake, J.M. Global patterns of zoonotic disease in mammals. *Trends Parasitol.* **2016**, *32*, 565–577. [CrossRef]
33. United Nations Department of Economic and Social Affairs, Population Division, World Population Prospects 2019. Highlights (ST/ESA/SER.A/423). Available online: https://population.un.org/wpp/Publications/Files/WPP2019_Highlights.pdf (accessed on 10 August 2019).
34. Garske, T.; Yu, H.; Peng, Z.; Ye, M.; Zhou, H.; Cheng, X.; Wu, J.; Ferguson, N. Travel patterns in China. *PLoS ONE* **2011**, *6*, e16364. [CrossRef]
35. Goldsmid, J.M. *The Travel Bug*; Occ. Paper No 17; University of Tasmania: Hobart, Australia, 1979.
36. Angelo, K.M.; Kozarsky, P.E.; Ryan, E.T.; Chen, L.H.; Sotir, M.J. What proportion of international travellers acquire a travel-related illness? A review of the literature. *J. Travel Med.* **2017**, *24*. [CrossRef]
37. Australian Bureau of Statistics. Overseas Arrivals and Departures, Australia, July 2019 cat. no. 3401.0. Available online: https://www.abs.gov.au/ausstats/abs@.nsf/featurearticlesbyCatalogue/A5438F2F06B39A8FCA258493001E8822?OpenDocument (accessed on 5 September 2019).
38. Maloney, S.A.; Weinberg, M. Prevention of infectious diseases among international pediatric travelers: Considerations for clinicians. *Semin. Pediatr. Infect. Dis.* **2004**, *15*, 137–149. [CrossRef]
39. Leder, K.; Torresi, J.; Libman, M.D.; Cramer, J.P.; Castelli, F.; Schlagenhauf, P.; Wilder-Smith, A.; Wilson, M.E.; Keystone, J.S.; Schwartz, E.; et al. GeoSentinel surveillance of illness in returned travelers, 2007–2011. *Ann. Intern. Med.* **2013**, *158*, 456–468. [CrossRef]
40. Harvey, K.; Esposito, D.H.; Han, P.; Kozarsky, P.; Freedman, D.O.; Plier, D.A.; Sotir, M.J. Surveillance for travel-related disease—GeoSentinel surveillance system, United States, 1997–2011. *MMWR Surveill. Summ.* **2013**, *62*, 1–23.
41. Leung, D.T.; LaRocque, R.C.; Ryan, E.T. Travel Medicine. *Ann. Intern. Med.* **2018**, *168*, ITC1–ITC16. [CrossRef]
42. James, S.L.; Abate, D.; Abate, K.H.; Abay, S.M.; Abbafati, C.; Abbasi, N.; Abbastabar, H.; Abd-Allah, F.; Abdela, J.; Abdelalim, A.; et al. Global, regional, and national incidence, prevalence, and years lived with disability for 354 diseases and injuries for 195 countries and territories, 1990–2017: A systematic analysis for the Global Burden of Disease Study 2017. *Lancet* **2018**, *392*, 1789–1858. [CrossRef]

43. Garcia, H.H.; Nash, T.E.; Del Brutto, O.H. Clinical symptoms, diagnosis, and treatment of neurocysticercosis. *Lancet Neurol.* **2014**, *13*, 1202–1215. [CrossRef]
44. Roman, G.; Sotelo, J.; Del Brutto, O.; Flisser, A.; Dumas, M.; Wadia, N.; Botero, D.; Cruz, M.; Garcia, H.; De Bittencourt, P.R.M.; et al. A proposal to declare neurocysticercosis an international reportable disease. *Bull. World Health Organ.* **2000**, *78*, 399–406.
45. Hunter, E.; Cliff, M.; Armstrong, M.; Manji, H.; Jäger, H.R.; Chiodini, P.; Brown, M. Active neurocysticercosis at the Hospital for Tropical Diseases, London: A clinical case series. *Trans. R. Soc. Trop. Med. Hyg.* **2018**, *112*, 326–334. [CrossRef] [PubMed]
46. Goldsmid, J. *The Deadly Legacy: Australian History and Transmissible Disease*; (No. 3); New South Wales University Press: Kensington, Australia, 1988; p. 115.
47. Beard, T.C. Hydatid control: A problem in health education. *Med. J. Aust.* **1969**, *2*, 456–459. [CrossRef]
48. Beard, T.C.; Bramble, A.J.; Middleton, M.J. *Eradication in Our Lifetime: A Log Book of the Tasmanian Hydatid Control Programs, 1962–1996*; Department of Primary Industries, Water and Environment: Hobart, Tasmania, Australia, 2001.
49. Gemmell, M.A. Australasian contributions to an understanding of the epidemiology and control of hydatid disease caused by *Echinococcus granulosus*—Past, present and future. *Int. J. Parasitol.* **1990**, *20*, 431–456. [CrossRef]
50. Jenkins, D.J. *Echinococcus granulosus* in Australia, widespread and doing well! *Parasitol. Int.* **2006**, *55*, S203–S206. [CrossRef] [PubMed]
51. Andrews, J.R.; Ainsworth, R.; Abernethy, D. *Trichinella pseudospiralis* in humans: Description of a case and its treatment. *Trans. R. Soc. Trop. Med. Hyg.* **1994**, *88*, 200–203. [CrossRef]
52. Andrews, J.R.; Ainsworth, R.; Pozio, E. Nematodes in human muscle. *Parasitol. Today* **1997**, *12*, 488–489. [CrossRef]
53. Andrews, J.R.H.; Bandi, C.; Pozio, E.; Morales, M.G.; Ainsworth, R.; Abernethy, D. Identification of *Trichinella pseudospiralis* from a human case using random amplified polymorphic DNA. *Am. J. Trop. Med. Hyg.* **1995**, *53*, 185–188. [CrossRef] [PubMed]
54. Spratt, D.M.; Beveridge, I.; Andrews, J.R.; Dennett, X. *Haycocknema perplexum* ng, n. sp. (Nematoda: Robertdollfusidae): An intramyofibre parasite in man. *Syst. Parasitol.* **1999**, *43*, 123–131. [CrossRef]
55. Vos, L.J.; Robertson, T.; Binotto, E. *Haycocknema perplexum*: An emerging cause of parasitic myositis in Australia. *Commun. Dis. Intell. Q. Rep.* **2016**, *40*, E496–E499. [PubMed]
56. Koehler, A.V.; Leung, P.; McEwan, B.; Gasser, R.B. Using PCR-Based Sequencing to Diagnose *Haycocknema perplexum* Infection in Human Myositis Case, Australia. *Emerg. Infect. Dis.* **2018**, *24*, 2368–2370. [CrossRef] [PubMed]
57. Basuroy, R.; Pennisi, R.; Robertson, T.; Norton, R.; Stokes, J.; Reimers, J.; Archer, J. Parasitic myositis in tropical Australia. *Med. J. Aust.* **2008**, *188*, 254–256. [PubMed]
58. Roth, J.A.; Galyon, J.; Stumbaugh, A. Causes and consequences of emerging and exotic diseases of animals: Role of the veterinarian. *Vet. Microbiol. Prev. Med. Publ.* **2010**, *91*, 10–17. Available online: https://lib.dr.iastate.edu/vmpm_pubs/91/ (accessed on 27 November 2019).
59. Spratt, D.M.; Beveridge, I. Wildlife parasitology in Australia: Past, present and future. *Aust. J. Zool.* **2019**, *66*, 286–305.
60. Kettlewell, J.S.; Bettiol, S.S.; Davies, N.; Milstein, T.; Goldsmid, J.M. Epidemiology of giardiasis in Tasmania: A potential risk to residents and visitors. *J. Travel Med.* **1998**, *5*, 127–130. [CrossRef]
61. Bettiol, S.S.; Kettlewell, J.S.; Davies, N.J.; Goldsmid, J.M. Giardiasis in native marsupials of Tasmania. *J. Wildl. Dis.* **1997**, *33*, 352–354. [CrossRef]
62. Kille, P.; Field, D.; Bailey, B.; Blaxter, M.; Morrison, N.; Snape, J.; Turner, S.; Viant, M. NERC Environmental 'Omics Strategy'. Available online: https://nerc.ukri.org/research/funded/programmes/omics/neomics-report/ (accessed on 5 September 2019).
63. Goldsmid, J.M.; Sullivan, P. Malaria in Tasmania 1987–1992. *J. Travel Med.* **1994**, *1*, 55–56. [CrossRef] [PubMed]
64. Ashley, E.A.; Phyo, A.P. Drugs in development for malaria. *Drugs* **2018**, *78*, 861–879. [CrossRef] [PubMed]
65. Laurens, M.B. RTS, S/AS01 vaccine (Mosquirix™): An overview. *Hum. Vaccin. Immunother.* **2019**, *22*, 1–10. [CrossRef] [PubMed]

66. Suder, E.; Furuyama, W.; Feldmann, H.; Marzi, A.; de Wit, E. The vesicular stomatitis virus-based Ebola virus vaccine: From concept to clinical trials. *Hum. Vaccin. Immunother.* **2018**, *14*, 2107–2113. [CrossRef] [PubMed]
67. Ganten, D.; Silva, J.G.; Regateiro, F.; Jafarian, A.; Boisjoly, H.; Flahault, A.; Canny, B.; Auler, J.O., Jr.; Kickbusch, J.; Heldmann, J.; et al. Science Has to Take Responsibility 10 Years World Health Summit—The Road to Better Health for All. *Front. Public Health* **2018**, *6*, 314. [CrossRef]
68. Havemann, M.; Bösner, S. Global Health as "umbrella term"—A qualitative study among Global Health teachers in German medical education. *Glob. Health* **2018**, *14*, 32. [CrossRef]
69. Banta, J.E. From international health to global health. *J. Community Health* **2001**, *26*, 73–76. [CrossRef]
70. Jain, S.C. Global health: Emerging frontier of international health. *Asia Pac. J. Public Health* **1991**, *5*, 112–114. [CrossRef]
71. Rabinowitz, P.M.; Natterson-Horowitz, B.J.; Kahn, L.H.; Kock, R.; Pappaioanou, M. Incorporating one health into medical education. *BMC Med. Educ.* **2017**, *17*, 45. [CrossRef]
72. Whitmee, S.; Haines, A.; Beyrer, C.; Boltz, F.; Capon, A.G.; de Souza, B.F.; Ezeh, A.; Frumkin, H.; Gong, P.; Head, P.; et al. Safeguarding human health in the Anthropocene epoch: Report of the Rockefeller Foundation-Lancet Commission on planetary health. *Lancet* **2015**, *386*, 1973–2028. [CrossRef]
73. Bradley, D.J. The scope of Travel Medicine: An introduction to the Conference on International Travel Medicine. In *Travel Medicine, Proceedings of the First Conference on International Travel Medicine, Zürich, Switzerland, 5–8 April 1988*; Steffen, R., Lobel, H.O., Haworth, J., Bradley, D.J., Eds.; Springer: Berlin/Heidelberg, Germany, 1989; pp. 1–596.

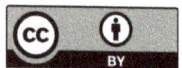

© 2020 by the authors. Licensee MDPI, Basel, Switzerland. This article is an open access article distributed under the terms and conditions of the Creative Commons Attribution (CC BY) license (http://creativecommons.org/licenses/by/4.0/).

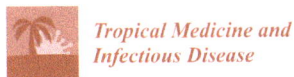

Commentary

The Importance of Understanding Social and Cultural Norms in Delivering Quality Health Care—A Personal Experience Commentary

Ahmed S. Latif

Public Health Physician, Formerly Professor of Medicine and Dean of College of Health Sciences, University of Zimbabwe, Harare, Zimbabwe; aslatif@gmail.com

Received: 16 January 2020; Accepted: 31 January 2020; Published: 5 February 2020

Abstract: The objectives of this paper are to provide a review of the author's personal experiences working in culturally diverse environments and to emphasize the importance of recognizing the social determinants of health. While some determinants of health are modifiable others are not, in addition it is emphasized that cultural safety in delivering health care is crucial if services provided are to be appropriate and acceptable to health care seekers. Cultural sensitivity is needed if one is to make a change in health outcomes in culturally diverse environments. The development and delivery of culturally safe services is more acceptable to community members and is important if a difference is to be made in health inequities. Training in delivering culturally safe services should include both theoretical and practical components. Practical training should be conducted under supervision in remote settings so that trainees appreciate what their clients experience on a daily basis. Culturally "unsafe" clinical service has serious adverse effects. This commentary discusses the above factors and provides example cases from the author's own career of where such factors have affected the health of individuals or groups.

Keywords: social determinants of health; cultural safety in health service delivery; cultural competency

---

Key Messages:

- There are a number of social determinants of health, some of these are modifiable while others such genetic make-up, gender and age are not.
- All health workers should receive education on the specific needs of their patients based on their culture, and, should understand that in a multi-cultural society, approaches to health delivery vary when dealing with patients differing cultures.
- In order for health care services to be effective they need to be both appropriate and acceptable and should be delivered by skilled and competent health care workers.
- Cultural awareness and cultural competency are required for cultural safety.
- Training for delivering culturally safe health care should include both theoretical and practical components.
- Not providing culturally safe services may result in serious adverse outcomes.

1. Introduction

In the early days of our own training, more than 50 years ago, we were made to learn of these factors. A number of texts by the very distinguished and respected Professor Michael Gelfand [1–3] were available. We were taught that "unless you approach your patients with understanding you will fail to win them over and as a result you will often be unable to cure them." This is quoted in a review of the publication in the Journal of the American Medical Association in 1964 [4]. As medical students, we took part in the "Medical Anthropology" described in the book, and, as part of this we visited remote communities in Zimbabwe (then Rhodesia) and learnt how traditional practitioners delivered health care to clients that consulted with them for their needs. More recent publications are also available, and a paper by Professor John Goldsmid is referenced here [5]. Professor Goldsmid emphasizes that human behaviour and cultural practices can have a profound effect on the range and prevalence of diseases suffered by communities and that human behaviour is the forgotten factor in disease prevalence and transmission.

My training in medicine was in Zimbabwe. After graduation in 1969, I worked as an intern, senior house officer, and a general practitioner before specializing in internal medicine and sexual health. I worked as a medical officer in the Harare City Health Department where I introduced the concept of the syndromic management of sexually transmitted infections. After specializing I joined the Department of Medicine of the University of Zimbabwe Medical School where I was involved in teaching undergraduates and postgraduates and conducting research and other academic activities. During this time I also worked as a consultant for the World Health Organization and was able to visit numerous countries where I was involved in training doctors and health staff and develop and set up programs for the management and control of sexually transmitted infections (STIs) and Human Immunodeficiency Virus (HIV) infection. I became Professor of Medicine at the University of Zimbabwe College of Medicine and later became Dean of the College of Medicine. Following this I took up an appointment as Public Health Medical Officer with the Department of Health of the Northern Territory in Australia and was based in Alice Springs, developing and implementing STI control activities. This provided me the opportunity to work Indigenous Aboriginal Communities in the Northern Territory of Australia and to learn the customs and needs of the local communities. In 2009, I accepted the post of Medical Director of an Aboriginal Community Controlled Health Organization in the Northern Territory, providing comprehensive primary health care and population health.

In order to improve the health status of an individual, the health status of the population in which the individual lives and works needs to be improved. Population health is defined as health outcomes of a group of individuals. Population health focuses on specific populations looking at a broad range of factors that affect health. These factors are known as social determinants of health. The World Health Organization lists the following factors that influence the health and well-being of individuals [6]:

- Income and social status
- Level of education
- Physical environment—including safe housing, clean air, safe water, healthy workplaces and healthy communities
- Social support networks—including support from family, friends and community, and, effect of individual behaviour
- Culture, customs and traditions
- Genetics—having a predisposition for some diseases and abnormalities
- Access to health services
- Gender of the individual—some illnesses are more frequent in males than females and vice versa

It is important that all trainees in the health service delivery area are taught that the health of their clients is affected by these factors and that without addressing these aspects the client's health may not improve or their problem will re-occur.

The importance of alternative medical systems cannot be over-emphasized. Depending on the region, country or continent, the public will seek care in alternative health systems. Hence the need to understand both what exists, and, what the health seeking behaviour of individuals is. In some countries in Southern Africa, the traditional healers play an important role in managing clients with chronic conditions and of conditions which suddenly develop without an obvious cause. An example of this is when the epidemic of HIV infection and AIDS started especially at the time (early in epidemic) when the cause of AIDS had not been established and no curative treatment was available. Illness may be "blamed" on misfortune or witchcraft and bad spirits, and hence clients would seek help in the alternative sector [7]. In many societies, the concept of disease origin is not completely understood by some of the populace, an example of this being the aetiology of disease [8]. The concept of the role of "invisible" pathogens and organisms, treatable or not, is not fully understood and requires a great deal of general education.

Box 1

> **Example Case 1**
> Early during the course of the outbreak of HIV infection and AIDS in Zimbabwe, before the etiologic agent, Human T Cell Lymphotropic Virus Type 3 (HTLV3 later the nomenclature changed and the etiologic agent was called the human immunodeficiency virus (HIV) was identified, we were faced with patients presenting with symptoms and signs of AIDS-associated conditions such as generalized lymphadenopathy, wasting, opportunistic infections and generalized aggressive Kaposi Sarcoma. In informing patients that there was no known cause for the condition, we inadvertently encouraged patients to seek care in the alternate sector. Later, when the etiologic agent was identified and patients were told that there was no known cure for the infection made patients more steadfast in seeking the help of traditional practitioners known as Ngangas. The services of the traditional practitioners were acceptable to care seekers who felt assured that they could be cured as they had always consulted with them from their early childhood days. Unfortunately, the Ngangas did not have a cure for this devastating infection which took the lives of thousands of infected persons. In the early days of the HIV epidemic, we had extensive discussions with traditional healers in Zimbabwe and even encouraged them to take part in some well-designed research activities.

The determinants of health are numerous. Some of these are non-modifiable, while others may be altered to the beneficial effects of individuals and communities. Non-modifiable determinants include age, gender, genetic make-up and family history. These are ingrained factors and are not modifiable. Modifiable determinants of health include: education, employment, financial income and social status, physical environment both at work and at leisure, housing and social environment, healthy childhood development, culture and personal and community practices, and availability of health services and social support [9–11].

2. Population Health and Public Health

Population health focusses on specific communities and populations to determine factors that influence health. These factors include the social determinants of health listed above. While population health focuses on specific populations or communities to improve the social and economic well-being as a whole, public health is the organized effort to keep persons and communities healthy and disease-free and to prevent injury, illness and premature death [12]. Constituents of public health include health protection, health surveillance, disease prevention, injury prevention, and health promotion. Population health and public health are closely related and work together hand-in-hand.

In providing health care it is important to understand that health services should at all times be accessible as well as acceptable.

It should however be noted that health care systems alone cannot improve population health without reducing the population's health and social inequities. A number of studies have shown that population health can improve if social needs are addressed and social conditions are improved [13].

The health of the individual and therefore of the community health is influenced by a number of complex factors that include: provision of acceptable, accessible and appropriate health care, individual and community health behaviours, physical and social environment, socioeconomic status, and public policy. These are all inter-related:

- Risky behaviours such as unhealthy diet and physical inactivity are linked with chronic diseases, but these risk factors depend on the community environment as people can only choose healthy options if these are available, and if the choices they make are safe.
- Socioeconomic status has a great influence on health as having the resources allows people to afford medical care, nutritious foods, and decent housing.

Public policy influences all of these aspects as it addresses education, employment and inequities, both nationally and locally, in both the private and public sectors.

In developing and providing health care services it is important to keep in mind a number factors including whether the service being provided is appropriate for the community receiving the service, whether the service is accessible, and finally whether the service is acceptable. These aspects need careful consideration and will determine whether the services will be used by the community. Considerations include opening hours for the service, gender distribution of staff providing services, distance of service from where people live, availability of transport, and costs for seeking the service.

3. Cultural Awareness

The health care provider's cultural awareness is their understanding of the differences between themselves and people from other backgrounds, especially relating to differences in values and attitudes [14]. It is important to understand that a lack of awareness can lead to bad or poor decision-making and poor outcomes for persons that we are supposedly providing help. Cultural awareness helps to reduce the chances of making bad decisions and increases the chance of us making appropriate and acceptable decisions.

Training in Cultural Awareness

It is important that health care providers have an understanding of what may or may not be culturally acceptable to the clients that they are dealing with. A number of different approaches are available in delivering cultural awareness training. Training may be theoretical or practical, however, ideally both these components are necessary in order to ensure that the trainee is well-equipped in delivering high quality, acceptable care. Theoretical training may be used to sensitize trainees in being aware that their clients' needs and beliefs may be different from what they themselves understand. It trains care providers in having an open mind and to ask their patients the right questions in the most acceptable way. Practical training is necessary to ensure that trainees consult with their patients and deliver care in an appropriate and acceptable way.

A number of training programs are available including face-to-face training, reading, and on-line courses. Some educational institutes have developed questionnaires that can be used when consulting with patients. Health care providers can ask a set of questions in order to determine the patients' social status and figure out what the role of social determinants may play in their health. The American Academy of Family Practice has developed a screening tool to determine whether the patient has a need for social services such as housing, food security, transportation, and to determine the patient's personal safety issues [15]. This short questionnaire may be used to determine whether the patient has modifiable social determinants of health. Training should aim to make health care providers competent in delivering culturally appropriate health care [16].

However, short training courses may not be sufficient for the delivery of culturally appropriate and culturally safe health care as shown in the Closing the Gap Report of The Australian Institute of Health and Welfare (AIHW) of the Australian Government published in 2015. This report states that cultural competency improves accessibility and effectiveness of healthcare for Indigenous people, however, in Australia, there is no coherent approach to embedding cultural competence in health services and that there is little evidence of how best to improve culturally competent healthcare delivery to Indigenous Australians [17].

Working in remote communities in the Northern Territory of Australia has been a great learning experience as well as an eye-opener. Firstly because of the remoteness of communities it is always difficult to recruit health staff. And secondly, health staff recruited tend to remain a short while. This requires that training needs to be repeated often. Staff obtained through recruitment agencies may come from all over Australia and even overseas. Recruitment agencies endeavor to train new recruits in cultural competency but of necessity the method of training is the short course type or even simply on-line. This may provide the trainee with an overview but does not provide them with a hands-on type experience. Hence, health organizations recruiting new staff need to develop their own cultural awareness and competency training. This is fine for long-term recruits but as often happens such recruits come in on short contracts. There is, therefore, a need for cultural awareness and competency training to take place during the undergraduate training of students in all disciplines of health.

Box 2

Example Case 2
The lack of cultural awareness by health care providers can lead to non-acceptance of services provided. This is particularly important in providing sexual health care services. In this situation the gender of health care providers should match the gender of care seeker. When providing services for women it is important for the patient to be seen by a female care provider, and similarly when dealing with male clients the provider should be male. In my own experience both in Africa and in Australia, I found that it is better not to raise certain topics when managing patients of the opposite gender. In fact, I realized that some words are considered taboo when uttered by a male during a discussion with a female patient. Being aware of such sensitivity is important if trust is to be gained from your patients. In situations where it is necessary for the patient to be provided the information, I found that by bringing in another female staff member (with the permission of the patient) to talk to the patient in my absence was preferable and more acceptable to the patient. When I was in formal non-clinical meetings with senior executive staff, I was advised by female executive staff members that they would prefer to have discussions on sexual health topics with a female clinician.
Being culturally aware is to have the knowledge and being culturally competent is to practice in a culturally safe manner.

In order for health care services to be effective, health care that is provided needs to be acceptable to the people served. Health care services will be considered acceptable to people if they are delivered in a culturally appropriate manner. The provision of culturally appropriate care requires an understanding of the social life and customs of the population served. In Zimbabwe and many other developing countries in Africa the medical teaching curricula include theoretical and practical training in this field. Medical students are exposed to the structure and function of traditional healing process and to social and cultural norms by having to live and learn in remote communities during their undergraduate training. During such remote placements a group of students would live in the community for periods of 3–4 weeks with their medical school supervisors and become involved in dealing with medical problems that the community has to face. Depending on the stage of the students' medical training, they are required to provide solutions to real-life or hypothetical problems that a community may face. This form of community orientated problem-based teaching takes place annually addressing different scenarios. In this way students learn to work with leaders and community decision makers including elders and traditional practitioners in dealing with major and minor issues that the community faces. The medical curriculum of the University of Zimbabwe College of Medicine is a comprehensive integrated curriculum which allows students to learn through problem solving exercises. Each year of their undergraduate training, students spend to three weeks in remote communities with supervisors and are exposed to local problems. They will observe and, where possible, assist the local community in dealing with existing problems and help identify causes of such problems as well as how to manage them locally. Medical students are placed in different communities in each of their placements.

With this approach students learn of the social, economic and physical environment that their patients come from and also get an understanding of the person's individual characteristics and behaviours. Importantly, in addition the student is able to identify the social support networks available to patients locally. It is well understood that greater support from families, friends, and communities is linked to better health. Studying during remote placements allows students to learn the culture, customs, traditions, and the beliefs of the family and community, all of which affect health.

4. Cultural Safety

A number of different terms have been used to describe the provision of acceptable and appropriate care for persons belonging to cultures that differ from that of the care provider. While these are processes that lead to the provision of acceptable care, cultural safety is the outcome of these processes. With patient safety in mind, the concept of cultural safety is defined by the Australian Health Practitioner Regulation Authority (AHPRA) as the individual and institutional knowledge, skills, attitudes and competencies needed to deliver optimal health care for Aboriginal and Torres Strait Islander Peoples [18]. The Cultural Safety covers a large number of terms currently used interchangeably, including: cultural awareness, cultural competence, cultural capability and proficiency, cultural respect, cultural security, cultural appropriateness, cultural understanding, and cultural responsiveness. These are all important in leading to the main outcome of cultural safety. In its statement AHPRA states "that patient safety for Aboriginal and Torres Strait Islander Peoples is the norm and that patient safety includes the inextricably linked elements of clinical and cultural safety, and this link must be defined by Aboriginal and Torres Strait Islander Peoples".

The importance of cultural safety cannot be over-emphasized especially since Australia is composed of a multi-cultural society in which everyone has the right to be treated with respect and dignity and this is crucial when delivering health care. Culturally safe health care delivery is crucial in attempting to close the gap in health outcomes in all communities.

Not providing a culturally safe service may lead to ill health such as low utilization of available services, non-compliance with referrals or prescribed interventions, reluctance in interacting with service providers, anger, and, dissatisfaction with tools and interventions used in the dominant culture [19].

In remote Aboriginal communities it is often stated that persons with chronic diseases are often not compliant with medicines prescribed for their illnesses. However, the reason for non-compliance may well be attributed to the lack of cultural awareness and competence of health practitioners, and this matter should be addressed.

5. Conclusions

Individual health is determined by a number of factors. While some of these factors are engrained in the individual and are not modifiable, the majority of determinants are modifiable. As health care providers it is our duty to identify the modifiable risk factors and initiate steps to modify these. Health is affected by the place the patient lives in, where they work, as well as where they are schooled. It is known that by eating well and staying active, not smoking, and seeking care when needed all influence health outcomes. Access to social and economic opportunities and availability of resources as well as availability of clean water and air also affect health and wellbeing [20]. Hence, addressing the social determinants health is important in achieving the goal of closing the gap in health inequities.

Training in cultural awareness and competency may be theoretical or practical. Theoretical training raises cultural awareness and provides guidance on its various different components and how to approach the topic. However, practical training provides the trainee with the experience necessary to provide culturally appropriate care and sensitizes the trainee on the multifactorial nature of the social determinants that the patient is surrounded by. Training in the classroom situation is not sufficient to reach the goals of provision of culturally appropriate care. By learning within the community, trainees are able to appreciate the fuller extent of the root causes of their patients' ill health, and by understanding these, the care provider is able to "manage" their patient in a complete and comprehensible way. Cultural competency training should be a mandatory requirement for all trainees in every branch of the health field.

Funding: This research received no external funding.

Conflicts of Interest: The author declares no conflict of interest.

References

1. Gelfand, M. *Medicine and Custom in Africa*; E and S Livingstone: Edinburgh, Scotland, UK, 1964.
2. Gelfand, M. The Sick African. In *A Clinical Study*; With a Foreword by Col. A. P. Martin; Post Graduate Press and Stewart Printing Co. (Pty.) Ltd.: Capetown, South Africa, 1944.
3. Gelfand, M. The principles and the practice of the Nanga. *Cent. Afr. J. Med.* **1981**, *27*, 71–73. [PubMed]
4. Callaway, W. Medicine and Custom in Africa. *JAMA* **1964**, *190*, 559. [CrossRef]
5. Goldsmid, J. Custom, culture and health in the tropics. Chapter 4. In *Primer of Tropical Medicine*; Goldsmid, J.M., Leggatt, P.A., Eds.; Australasian College of Tropical Medicine Web Edition: Townsville, Australia, 2013; Available online: https://www.tropmed.org/publications/primer-of-tropical-medicine/ (accessed on 4 January 2020).
6. World Health Organization. Health Impact Assessment—The Determinants of Health. Geneva, Switzerland, 2013; Available online: https://www.who.int/hia/evidence/doh/en/ (accessed on 4 January 2020).
7. Kleinman, A.K. Patients and healers in the context of culture. In *An Exploration of the Border-Land between Anthropology, Medicine and Psychiatry*; University of California Press: Berkeley, CA, USA, 1980.
8. Cockburn, A. Where did our infectious diseases come from? In *Health and Disease in Tribal Societies*; Hugh-Jones, P., Ed.; Elsevier: Amsterdam, The Netherlands, 1977; pp. 103–113.
9. US Office of Disease Prevention and Health Promotion. Available online: https://www.healthypeople.gov/ (accessed on 4 January 2020).
10. World Health Organization. Available online: https://www.who.int/social_determinants/en/ (accessed on 4 January 2020).
11. National Association of Aboriginal Community Controlled Organizations (NACCHO). Available online: https://nacchocommunique.com/social-determinants-of-health/ (accessed on 4 August 2019).
12. The Chief Public Health Officer's Report on the State of Public Health in Canada 2008—What is Public Health? Available online: https://www.canada.ca/en/public-health (accessed on 29 December 2019).
13. Woolf, S.H. Why Health Care Alone Cannot Improve Population Health and Reduce Health Inequities. *Ann. Fam. Med.* **2019**, *17*, 196–199. [CrossRef] [PubMed]
14. Cultural Awareness. Available online: https://www.collinsdictionary.com/dictionary/english/cultural-awareness (accessed on 4 January 2020).
15. Social Needs Screening Tool. Available online: https://www.aafp.org/dam/AAFP/documents/patient_care/everyone_project/patient-short-web.pdf (accessed on 2 January 2020).
16. *Cultural Competency in Health: A Guide for Policy, Partnerships and Participation*; NHMRC, 2006. Available online: https://www.nhmrc.gov.au/about-us/publications/cultural-competency-health (accessed on 15 January 2020).
17. Bainbridge, R.; McCalman, J.; Clifford, A.; Tsey, K.; For the Closing the Gap Clearinghouse. Cultural Competency in the Delivery of Health Services for Indigenous People. Available online: https://www.aihw.gov.au/reports/indigenous-australians/cultural-competency-in-the-delivery-of-health-services-for-indigenous-people (accessed on 4 January 2020).
18. Australian Health Practitioner Regulation Authority. Aboriginal and Torres Strait Islander Health Strategy—Statement of Intent. 2019. Available online: https://www.ahpra.gov.au/About-AHPRA/Aboriginal-and-Torres-Strait-Islander-Health-Strategy/Statement-of-intent.aspx (accessed on 15 January 2020).

19. Ball, J. Cultural Safety in Practice with Children, Families and Communities. Early Childhood Development Intercultural Partnerships. 2005. Available online: https://www.ecdip.org/culturalsafety/ (accessed on 30 January 2020).
20. Social Determinants of Health|Healthy People. 2020. Available online: https://www.healthypeople.gov/2020/topics-objectives/topic/social-determinants-of-health (accessed on 3 January 2020).

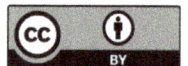

© 2020 by the author. Licensee MDPI, Basel, Switzerland. This article is an open access article distributed under the terms and conditions of the Creative Commons Attribution (CC BY) license (http://creativecommons.org/licenses/by/4.0/).

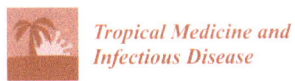

Review

Ternidens deminutus Revisited: A Review of Human Infections with the False Hookworm

Richard S. Bradbury

Slovak Tropical Institute, St. Elizabeth University, 81101 Bratislava, Slovakia; rbradbur76@gmail.com

Received: 18 June 2019; Accepted: 17 July 2019; Published: 18 July 2019

Abstract: *Ternidens deminutus*, the false hookworm of humans and non-human primates, represents a truly neglected intestinal helminth infection. The similarity of the eggs of this nematode to those of hookworm both presents a diagnostic challenge and a potential confounder in prevalence surveys of soil transmitted helminths (STH) in regions where *T. deminutus* is found. The helminth infects non-human primates throughout Africa and Asia, but reports of human infection are almost exclusively found in eastern and southern Africa. Historically, an infection prevalence up to 87% has been reported from some parts of Zimbabwe. Scarce reports of ternidensiasis have also been made in individuals in Suriname and one from Thailand. Little work has been performed on this parasite since the 1970s and it not known why human infection has not been reported more widely or what the current prevalence in humans from historically endemic areas is. This review serves to revisit this enigmatic parasite and provide detail to a modern audience of parasitologists on its history, clinical presentation, geographic distribution, life cycle, biology, morphology, diagnosis and treatment.

Keywords: *Ternidens*; ternidensiasis; false hookworm; hookworm; soil transmitted helminths; STH; helminth; zoonosis; human; primate

1. Introduction

The World Health Organization's (WHO) global target to eliminate morbidity due to soil-transmitted helminths in children by 2020 [1] has resulted in increased interest within the global health community towards the control of STH (the hookworms, *Ascaris lumbricoides* and *Trichuris trichiura*). This has included increased activity in the global surveillance of hookworm and other STH prevalence [2]. Surveillance activities in most countries still rely on microscopic detection and identification of eggs. Discrepancies between microscopy and PCR results in some of these surveys have highlighted the existence of human infecting helminths having eggs that may be morphologically confused with those of STH [3]. This has raised the need to revisit the intestinal helminths of humans that are historically known to occur at moderate to high prevalence in some populations and are having eggs morphologically similar to those of other STH.

Ternidens deminutus (the false hookworm) is one such helminth, with infected humans passing eggs that are easily confused with hookworm eggs. Surveys of human intestinal helminths in Zimbabwe during the 1970s revealed a prevalence of this parasite of up to 87% in some populations [4]. The remarkable similarity of *T. deminutus* eggs to those of hookworms often confounded previous surveys of hookworm prevalence in these regions [5]. Furthermore, *T. deminutus* infection has not been reported from humans in any surveillance studies for the past 25 years [6], nor in any individual case report since 2005 [7]. In areas where prevalence of this worm was historically high, such as southern Zimbabwe, this is likely due to misidentification of *T. deminutus* eggs as those of hookworms, rather than elimination of the parasite from these communities. It appears to be time to revisit *Ternidens* and to inform the current generation of parasitologists and epidemiologists of the existence, diagnosis and treatment of this neglected tropical disease.

Several countries, regions and cities referred to in this review have changed their names multiple times over the past one hundred years. To avoid confusion for readers, the place names current at the time of writing have been used throughout.

2. History

T. deminutus (nematoda: Strongylidae) is an intestinal helminth of primates, including humans, monkeys, gorillas and baboons in Africa and Asia (Table 1). The species was first described by Railliet and Henry (1905) [8] when reviewing two museum specimens taken at autopsy in 1865 by the French naval physician Moniester from the intestine of a patient native to Mozambique (but living on the island of Mayotte) who had died of anemia. Originally incorrectly identified as *Ancylostoma duodenale* by Moniester, Railliet and Henry differentiated the worms on the basis of morphology and described them as *Triodontophorus deminutus* [8]. In 1908, Turner found upon autopsy a number of female worms in the large intestine of two patients from Malawi who had died working in the mines of Johannesburg (South Africa). These worms were distinct from the *Necator americanus* specimens found in the same patient's small intestine, both in their morphology and that the site of infection was the large intestine. Leiper (1908) [9] examined these worms and identified them as *T. deminutus* [10]. The following year, Railliet and Henry (1909) [11] revised the taxonomy of the family *Strongylidae* and the name *Triodontophorus* was suppressed as a synonym for a new genus, *Ternidens*. Stannus sent a number of worms recovered post-mortem from the intestines of prisoners from Loma, Malawi to Leiper who identified them as *T. deminutus*, though these particular cases were not reported in the literature until they were communicated by Sandground in 1931 [12].

Infection in primates was first reported by Leiper, in a western lowland gorilla (*Gorilla gorilla gorilla*) taken from Gabon which died at the London zoological gardens. Between 1906 and 1937, infection was identified in numerous species of monkeys from Africa and Asia, as well as in a baboon (*Papio ursinus griseipes*) and a chimpanzee (*Pan troglodytes versus*) [13]. Smith, Fox and White (1908) [14] described a new worm, *Globocephalus macaci* in a pig-tailed monkey (*Macaca nemestrina nemestrina*) which died at the Philadelphia zoo, but this worm was considered to be *T. deminutus* by Sandground [12].

The significance of *T. deminutus* as a human pathogen became more widely recognized following the work of Sandground in Zimbabwe in the late 1920s [12,15]. Sandground first identified a novel and unusual helminth egg in the feces of an American medical missionary working in the Mount Selinda region of that country. He first considered this nematode as possibly belonging to the genera *Trichostongylus* or *Oesophagostomum*. However, on receipt of several fecal samples and adult worms taken from people in the immediate vicinity of the mission where the patient worked, the parasites were identified as *T. deminutus* [15].

In response to this finding, Sandground traveled to Southern Africa and carried out surveys for *T. deminutus* infection on workers at the City Deep Goldmine in Johannesburg, the Mount Selinda and Chikore regions of south east Zimbabwe, Livingstone in Zambia and the Gogoyo region and Maputo city regions of Mozambique. Based on results from the NaCl passive flotation technique, *Ternidens* infection prevalence of over 50% was reported from some regions, while in others few or no *T. deminutus* infections were identified. In Johannesburg, 15 of 503 individuals (3%) were found to be infected with *T. deminutus*, eleven of whom were from Mozambique, although some patients from the Eastern Cape and Gauteng region of South Africa were also found to be infected [15]. At Mt. Selinda, 112/190 (59%) of individuals tested harbored *T. deminutus*, either alone (n = 48) or in co-infection with hookworms (n = 64). At Chikore, 8/12 (67%) were infected, while at Gogoyo, 34/124 (27%) were infected, with all but one being co-infected with hookworms. No *T. deminutus* infections were found amongst 54 individuals in Livingstone. Of 323 individuals from many parts of Mozambique examined in Maputo, only one was infected with *Ternidens* [12]. At Mount Selinda, infection intensity of between 21 and one hundred individual worms was identified in some patients following treatment with carbon tetrachloride, terachloroethylene or a combination of these drugs with oil of chemopodium [12].

Following Sandground's work, Blackie reported that prevalence of *T. deminutus* infection was between 5.3% and 16% in various parts of Zimbabwe [16], while Van den Berghe (1934) [17] reported a prevalence of 15% in a survey of people in the Katanga region of the Democratic Republic of Congo. A single case was reported from Zambia by Blackie in 1932 [16] and from Mauritius in 1937 by Webb [18]. Forty-four adult worms were provided to the US Naval Medical School in 1947 by the Central Medical Laboratories in Maputo, Mozambique [13]. Several hookworm surveys in Zimbabwe by Gelfand between 1945 and 1965 failed to detect the parasite, which was later suggested as being possibly due to failure to differentiate the eggs from those of hookworm rather than due to its absence in the populations sampled [5].

Table 1. Reported non-human primate hosts of *Ternidens deminutus* and their geographic range.

Host name	Common name	Region
Cercocebus atys	Sooty mangabey	Africa
Cercopithecus ascanius schmidti	Red tailed monkey	Africa
Cercopithecus campbelli	Campbell's monkey	Africa
Cercopithecus cephus	Moustached guenon	Africa
Cercopithecus diana	Diana monkey	Africa
Cercopithecus mona	Mona monkey	Africa
Cercopithecus petaurista	Lesser spot-nosed monkey	Africa
Chlorocebus aethiops centralis	Grey monkey	Africa
Chlorocebus pygerythrus	Vervet (green) monkey	Africa
Gorilla gorilla gorilla	Western Gorilla	Africa
Macaca mulatta	Rhesus monkey	South East Asia and India
Macaca nemestrina nemestrina	Pig tailed macaque	South East Asia
Macaca nigra	Black macaque	South East Asia
Macaca radiata	Bonnet monkey	India
Macaca fascicularis fascicularis	Crab eating macaque	South East Asia
Pan troglodytes versus	Chimpanzee	Africa
Papio anubis	Olive baboon	Africa
Papio ursinus griseipes	Chacma baboon	Africa
Pongo pygmaeus	Bornean orang utan	South East Asia

3. Biology and Life Cycle

The closest relative to of the genus *Ternidens* is *Oesophagostomum* [19,20], another nodular intestinal worm affecting both humans and non-human primates in Africa and Asia. Only two species are currently recognized in the genus; *T. deminutus* and *Ternidens simiae*. *T. deminutus* has been reported in monkeys, baboons and humans in Africa and Asia (Table 1). The average size of *T. deminutus* adults in humans is larger than that of baboons [21]. *T. simiae* has been reported once from the gut of a monkey in Sulawesi, Indonesia [22], but could not be confirmed [23]. Genetic variations between *T. deminutus* from different monkey hosts has raised the possibility that several cryptic species may infect different host primates [19,20].

Infection of the definitive host may occur via oral ingestion of third stage (L3 filariform) larvae [24], which establish parasitism in the large intestine, particularly the colon, but also the cecum, compared to hookworms, which are primarily parasites of the duodenum. These L3 larvae are thought to then enter the intestinal mucosa, form nodules in which they mature to L4 larvae and then re-enter the lumen as adults to mate [12,24]. Based on observations of blood in the intestine of adult worms [21] combined with histochemical and biochemical analysis of the contents of worm guts [25] that adult worms possibly ingest blood. Whether they are true blood suckers or simply ingest blood oozing from lesions that they have created in the intestinal mucosa remains unclear [21].

Infections in human subjects examined by Goldsmid [26] found a mean worm load of 22.7 ± 5.9 worms per subject and a mean egg output of 494.4 ± 158.4 eggs per gram of feces, with a mean egg production of approximately 3500 and 7000 eggs/worm per day [26]. Eggs are passed with eight stage (rarely four stage) morulae in the feces [21]. The female:male ratio in both baboons and humans was 1:6 [26]. Eggs become fully mature 24 to 30 h after passage and the L1 (rhabditiform larvae) hatch after 48-72 h. The L1 rhabditiform larvae develop into L2 stage after two to three days at 29 °C. Development to L3 filariform larvae at this temperature takes eight to ten days [26]. The L3 larvae of *T. deminutus* appear to be relatively environmentally resistant. Sandground claimed to have revived larvae following three days of desiccation [12]. Experiments by Goldsmid found that approximately 4% of L3 larvae survived and recovered motility after 24 h of desiccation at 14 °C at 60% relative humidity. After 24 h in these desiccated conditions, no larvae survived [26]. The morphology of revived larvae following desiccation was greatly affected, with many losing their sheath, developing vacuoles in the cuticle and internal structures becoming unrecognizable [12,26], and thus the infectivity of such affected larvae is not reliable. Resistance to cold was also observed, with over 60% of 224 larvae surviving at 5 °C for ten days. Survival continued for 70 days, though the percentage of viable larvae rapidly declined by this time. No viable larvae were detected at 84 days. Larvae did not survive freezing at −5 °C for one hour [26]. As is seen with hookworm infection, the passage of *T. deminutus* eggs in feces shows a seasonal prevalence, with the highest rates of detection in Zimbabwe being during the Summer months, which are characterized by high temperatures and rainfall [20]. When 301 patients between the ages of 0–2 and >65 years of age were examined, egg output was greatest in patients between the ages of 7 and 35 years [20].

Although a direct life cycle is assumed, the failure of attempts to infect volunteers through ingestion of filariform larvae or by transdermal inoculation [12,15,16] also led to the proposal that an insect intermediate host may be involved in transmission [13,21,27]. Termites were suggested as such a possible host due to their being shared in the diet of both humans and monkeys in areas where human infection is common [28].

T. deminutus is thought to be a zoonosis acquired from non-human primates, although some "spillback" from humans to monkey populations may also occur in some areas [21]. Attempts to infect humans via oral ingestion of larvae cultured from a baboon by Sandground [12] were unsuccessful and some have suggested that humans may be the main host species [12,29]. The possible presence of multiple cryptic species might explain this controversy, with a human specific haplotype of the parasite existing alongside several host-specific non-human primate genotypes. This theory is supported by the analogous presence of several host-specific haplotypes, including a human-specific haplotype, in the genetically similar helminth species *Oesophagostomum bifurcum* [30]. The average size difference between adults in humans and baboons might support this, though such morphological variation in size between hosts is not uncommon in nematode species. This hypothesis would also explain the almost complete absence of human infections in Asia, despite the parasite being prevalent in non-human primates in the continent.

4. Geographic Distribution and Prevalence

Ternidens infections of monkeys, chimpanzees and baboons have been reported throughout sub-Saharan Africa and Asia (Table 1). Infections have thus far not been reported in new world primates. In humans, reports of infection have been almost exclusively from sub-Saharan Africa, with only one case report from Thailand and two from Suriname (Figure 1).

Human *T. deminutus* infections often occur in high prevalence foci, such as seen in several villages of Zimbabwe. In 1972, Goldsmid, undertook to revisit the work of Sandground [12] on *T. deminutus* and actively surveyed patients at the Harari Central Hospital in Harare, Zimbabwe. Of 5545 patients examined, 208 (3.75%) harbored infections [5]. Several further surveys in eastern and the central north of Zimbabwe (Bindura, Chiweshe, Burma Valley, Masvingo, Nyanga, Lundi, Maramba, Mount Selinda, Sabi Valley, Harare, Triangle and Mutare) by Goldsmid found a wide range of prevalence, between 0% and 87% (mean average 19%; median 9.2%), in humans. Of 32 baboons tested in Bikita and Marimba, over 70% were infected. No human cases were found in Kariba, in the North East Zambezi Valley area of the country [31]. A later survey in the Kadoma region of central Zimbabwe by Goldsmid found only 0.7% of 595 people infected [32]. In these surveys, Goldsmid applied the same NaCl passive flotation technique as Sandground had used in 1931 [12], with *T. deminutus* identification based on egg size and any difficult to differentiate eggs cultured by the Harada-Mori technique to allow definitive identification of the L3 larvae [5,31,32].

A survey of 4500 people from the Songea district of Tanzania found *T. deminutus* (identification based on egg size only, technique not stated) in 105 subjects [33]. In a report of 34 cases of intestinal helminthoma from Entebbe, Uganda in 1972, one case of *T. deminutus* helminthoma of the ileum was confirmed [34]. Two *Ternidens* infections, identified based on the morphology of the adult worms passed after treatment, in school children from Zimbabwe were reported in a study of the efficacy of albendazole as a hookworm treatment by Bradley in 1990 [35]. A further survey of people in the Burma Valley region of Zimbabwe in 1993 using quadruplicate Kato Katz examination, and identifying *T. deminutus* based on egg size alone, identified 5% as having *T. deminutus* infection [36].

Only one human *T. deminutus* case has been reported from Asia. This infection occurred in Thailand in 1983, but was not reported until 2002. A helminth was identified upon histology of an intestinal nodule taken from the colon of a 33 year old Thai female as an immature adult male *T. deminutus* [7]. In this case, the species identification and differentiation from the clinically and morphologically similar *Oesophagostomum* species was determined only by the width of the parasite in the histological section (300–500 µm; max 550 µm). This larger diameter was the only differentiating feature of this stage of *Ternidens* from *Oesophagostomum* in cross section and was the only feature used to make the species identification [7]. However, *Oesophagostomum* species in section may be up to 700 in diameter [37]. Furthermore, the diameter reported was below that reported for another *T. deminutus* (650 µm) infection in section, admittedly only measured in a single adult female [38]. Without other supporting molecular data, the only human case of human ternidensiasis reported from Asia may represent a misidentification of *Oesophagostomum* infection.

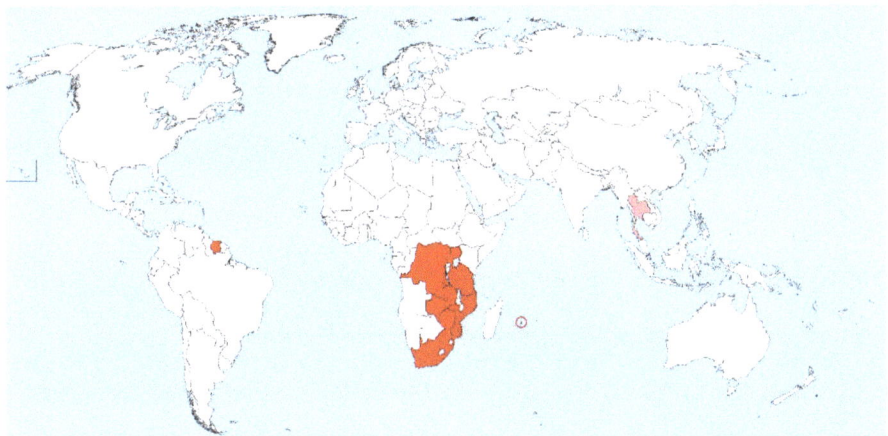

Figure 1. Map of the world showing countries (in red fill) where *Ternidens deminutus* infection in humans has been confirmed (red circle = Mauritius; pink fill = single case report, possible misidentification of *Oesophagostomum* infection).

Jozefsoon [6] reported two *T. deminutus* infections among 431 people belonging to a community of descendants of slaves brought from West Africa and living a traditional lifestyle in the southern interior of Suriname (South America). Identification was based on the morphologic identification of larvae in Harada-Mori culture, with the morphologic approaches described being reliable and the report therefore likely to be accurate. This report was particularly unusual as *T. deminutus* has not been reported from non-human primates on that continent. The people with *T. deminutus* infection in

Suriname may be the descendants of people that moved from West Africa, with the remnant worm population still circulating amongst this group [6]. Although it remains occasionally reported in non-human primates [39], no more cases of human *Ternidens* infection have been reported in the scientific literature since the two Suriname cases in 1994 [6]. Human *Ternidens* infections have almost certainly not disappeared since this time, rather, it seems likely that when encountered, they are being misidentified as hookworm or *Oesophagostomum*.

5. Morphology

The thin shelled eggs of *T. deminutus* superficially resemble those of hookworms (Figure 2). Eggs are also distinguished from those of hookworms by their larger size (70–94 μm × 40–60 μm) [21] and greater ratio of width to length (Figure 3) [12]. Eggs may have between four and 32 morulae, which will further develop into larvae within the egg and hatch.

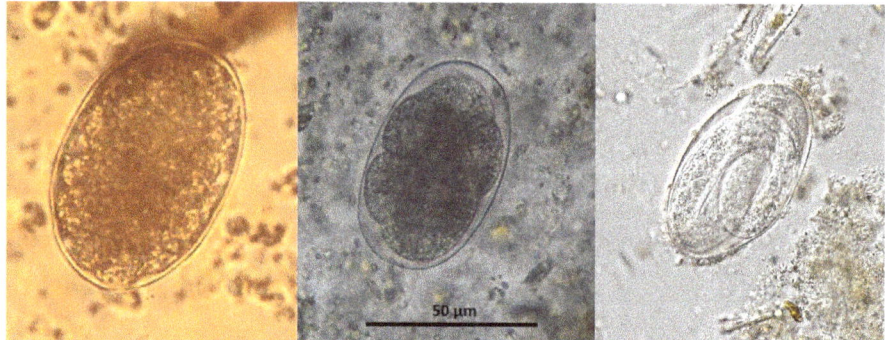

Figure 2. Eggs of *T. deminutus* (left – photographs courtesy of Emeritus Professor John Goldsmid), *Necator americanus* (middle - photograph by Richard Bradbury) and *Oesophagostomum* sp. (with larva developing within – photograph courtesy of CDC DPDx – https://www.cdc.gov/dpdx).

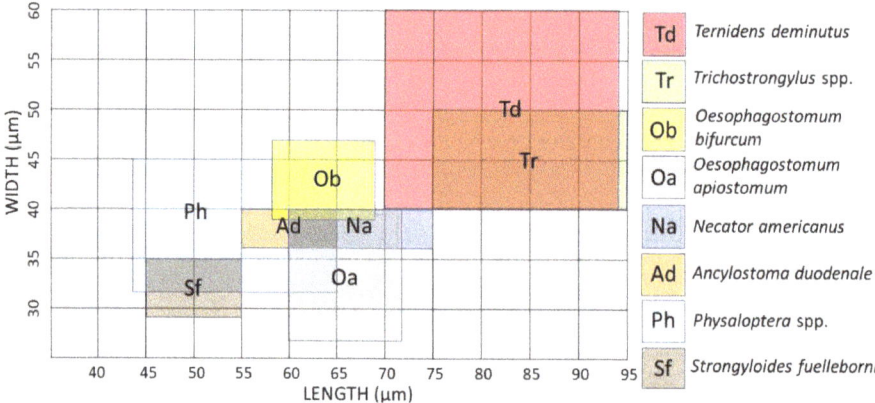

Figure 3. Size range comparison chart of hookworm-like eggs passed in human feces [21,40–42].

The first stage (L1) rhabditiform larvae of *T. deminutus* measure between 300 and 360 μm long by ~20 μm at the widest point [12] (Figure 4a). The cylindrical buccal cavity is 10.5 × 1.5 μm in length and breadth and the esophagus approximately 95 μm long. A refractile, spindle shaped genital primordium is 11.2 μm long. At the distal end, a long flagella-like tail reaches 70 μm in length [12]. L2 larvae are longer (620 μm) and wider (32 μm) with an esophagus 140 μm in length (Figure 4b). While these rhabditiform larvae appear similar to those of the hookworms and *Strongyloides stercoralis*, they may be differentiated by observing the combination of the long buccal cavity, prominent genital primordium, and longer tail.

The filariform (L3) stage larvae of *T. deminutus* (Figure 4c) are easily distinguished from other "hookworm-like" larvae derived from humans. This life stage measures between 630–730 μm long by 29–35 μm wide and is most distinguished by the palisade "zig-zag" appearance of the gut, shared with larvae of *Oesophagostomum*. The larval cuticle is distinctly striated and six minute, punctiform, papillae may be found on the head [12]. The head has an indentation at the entrance to the spear shaped remnant buccal cavity [21]. The esophagus measures 150-165 μm in length and is almost uniform in length and width, but for a slight bulge distally. The esophagus to intestine ration is approximately 1:3 [26]. Two elongate sphincter cells divide the esophagus from the intestine and the intestine is composed of at least ten pairs of large triangular cells which provide the palisade appearance of this organ. A genital primordium 15 μm long is found hugging the intestinal wall near the middle of the larva. The anus opens between 120-145 μm from the end of the tail [12]. The tail tapers to a fine point and the filamentous end of the sheath extends some distance further, appearing threadlike at the posterior extremity [6,12]. This morphologic appearance most closely resembles *Oesophagostomum* species L3 larvae, but the two may be differentiated by the greater overall length (702–950 μm), the "Y" shape of the remnant buccal cavity, the far wider and more prominent, rhabditoid esophageal bulb and the absence of sphincter cells between the esophagus and the intestine in *T. deminutus* L3 larvae. There is a much shorter distance from anus to the tip of the tail (45-88 μm) and the rounded tail of *Oesophagostomum* [6,40]. Jozefsoon [6] noted if the distance from the tip of the tail to the tip of the sheath is greater than the distance from the anus to the tip of tail, a larva is likely to represent an *Oesophagostomum* sp. and not *T. deminutus*.

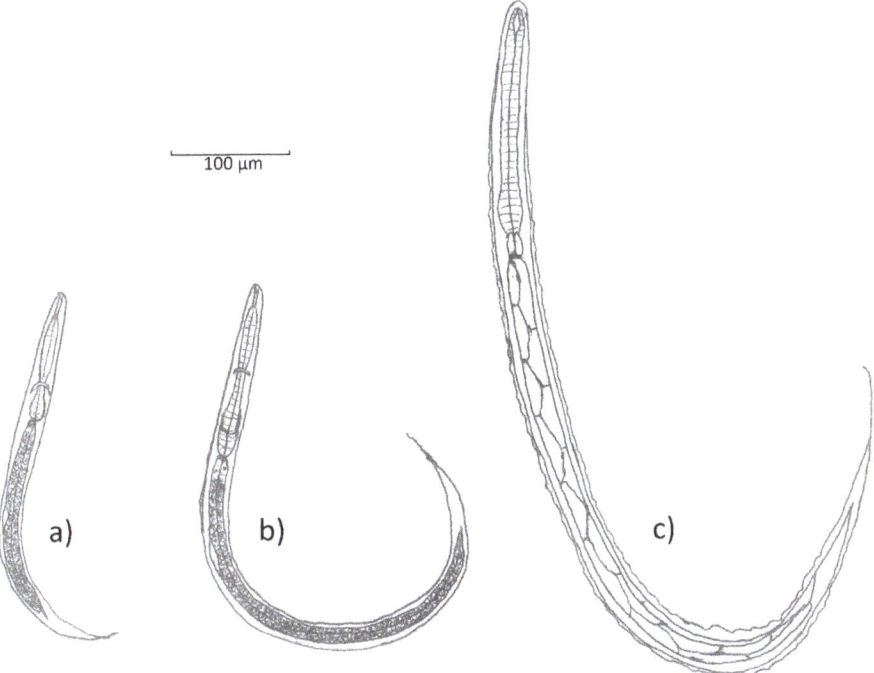

Figure 4. Line drawings showing the morphology of **a)** rhabditiform (L1) larva; **b)** rhabditiform (L2) larva and **c)** filariform (L3) larva of *Ternidens deminutus* (line drawings by Richard Bradbury).

Adult female *T. deminutus* from baboons are 5–12 mm in length (mean 8.60 ± 0.19 mm). Specimens from human hosts measure 9–17 mm in length (mean 11.56 ± 0.81 mm). Adult males are between 4.5–11 mm in length (mean 7.96 ± 0.21 mm) from baboons and 6–13 mm in length (mean 9.67 ± 0.66 mm) from human hosts. Specimens from humans appear to be darker in color than those from baboons [23]. Adult *Ternidens* are straight, unlike the curved appearance of adult hookworms. The cuticle is opaque and a transverse cuticular fold may be seen immediately distal to the buccal capsule. The entire cuticular surface has transverse striations. The large, swollen sub-globose buccal capsule contains an anteriorly facing mouth surrounded by a collar and 22–24 bristles of the corona radia (Figure 5). Four knob shaped sub median papillae and two lateral amphids are present on the anterior surface of the worm. On the base of the buccal capsule are three deep set teeth with two lateral and one central lamellae. The esophagus measures 525–840 (mean 739) μm in human derived worms and 511–837 (mean 727) μm in baboon derived worms. In females, the posterior tapers to a vulva and anus. The distance between the vulva and anus is 372–558 (mean 406) μm in human derived worms and 232–418 (mean 359) μm in baboon derived worms. In male worms, the anterior splays out into a cup shaped bursa consisting of rays encircling two copulatory spicules (Figure 5). A gubernaculum is present. The spicules measure 1116–1441 (mean 1267) μm in human derived worms and 1023–1302 (mean 1178) μm in baboon derived worms [23]. One description of the recovery of a rare deformed adult male *Ternidens* with bifurcated anterior was made by Lyons and Goldsmid in 1973 [43].

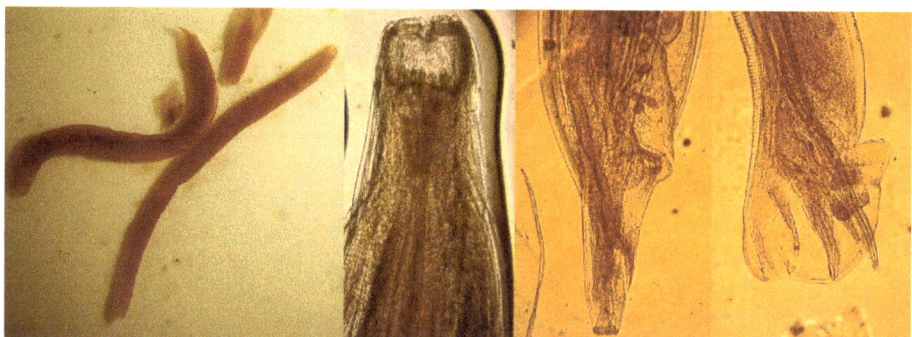

Figure 5. (left to right) adult *Ternidens deminutus* whole female and male worms from a human; anterior of an adult showing the buccal capsule, posterior of an adult female; posterior of an adult male showing copulatory bursa (photographs by Richard Bradbury).

6. Clinical Presentation

Ternidensiasis most commonly presents in a similar manner to oesophagostomiasis [19], with multiple intestinal abscesses, nodules or helminthomas of the large intestine [21]. Adult worms may also be found free in the intestinal lumen attached to the intestinal mucosa [26]. The clinical effects of infection have not been well studied. Infection appears to be asymptomatic in many cases. In some infections with heavy worm loads associated malaise, obstipation [13] and microcytic hypochromic anemia [21] have been reported. Due to the co-infections with other helminths and the poor nutritional condition of the participants involved in many studies, it is difficult to accurately discriminate the contribution of *Ternidens* infection to anemia as opposed to the effects of other chronic diseases and other parasitic infections.

7. Laboratory Diagnosis

The diagnosis of *Ternidens* has most commonly been undertaken by measurement of size and differentiated from hookworm based on the size of the eggs [21]. Eggs may be found in direct preparations, but recovery is increased by the use of techniques such as saturated salt flotation [12,24],

Kato Katz [34] and formalin-ethyl acetate sedimentation. Culture of larvae to L3 stage is recommended to allow definitive species identification [6]. Larval culture techniques such as Harada-Mori have been successfully employed to detect and identify *Ternidens* infections [24]. The Koga agar larval culture technique has not yet been applied the detection of *T. deminutus* but given the previous success of Harada-Mori technique, it appears likely that this method would also be successful. Recovery and identification of the adult worms on purgation or autopsy is the gold standard for diagnosis. No diagnostic PCR for the detection of *T. deminutus* has been developed thus far.

8. Treatment

As much of the work on *T. deminutus* was performed prior to the advent of benzimidazole derivative and macrocyclic lactone medications, there have been no controlled studies of the efficacy of modern anthelmintics commonly used in mass drug administration campaigns on *T. deminutus* infection. Historically, oil of chemopodium, carbon tetrachloride or tetrachloethylene were administered, but were ineffective [12,31]. Treatment with phenylene diisothyacyanate resulted in only a 22% cure rate and bephenium hydroxynapthoate an 87.5% cure rate [19]. Of the modern drugs available, Thiabendazole yielded a 90.5% cure rate, while Pyrantel pamoate cured 92% of cases [27]. One report has described the efficacy of albendazole when administered to two infected school children in Zimbabwe [34]. This suggests that albendazole may be a suitable treatment for *T. deminutus* infection, but more thorough trials involving albendazole, mebendazole and ivermectin with monitoring for a longer period following treatment would be advisable to comprehensively determine the most effective treatment for infections. In cases where *Ternidens* is causing a bowel helminthoma, surgical intervention may be indicated [34].

9. Conclusions

T. deminutus, the "false hookworm" has long been an enigmatic and often ignored intestinal helminth of humans. Studies into the worm and the disease caused by it have largely been undertaken by two enthusiastic and capable individuals, specifically John Sandground and John Goldsmid, while little attention was paid to this disease by other researchers. Ternidensiasis is a helminth infection of man capable of causing significant pathology in affected patients, including helminthomas and possibly iron deficiency anemia. No doubt the superficial similarity of the eggs to those of hookworm has led to it being misidentified as hookworm in areas of historically high prevalence, where it most likely remains a significant human helminthiasis and may confound the results of future STH prevalence surveys and control efforts. It is hoped that this paper will educate the modern STH and parasite diagnostics community on the existence and importance of *Ternidens* infection and will encourage further investigation by the community of unusual hookworm-like intestinal helminths into the future.

Funding: This research received no external funding.

Acknowledgments: This paper is dedicated to John Marsden Goldsmid, whose encouragement, mentoring and support were seminal in forming the author's career as a parasitologist.

Conflicts of Interest: The author declares no conflict of interest.

Disclaimer: Richard Bradbury is writing this paper in his personal capacity and in his capacity as a Visiting Professor of Public Health at the Slovak Tropical Institute, St. Elizabeth University, Bratislava, Slovakia.

References

1. World Health Organization. Intestinal Worms. 2019. Available online: www.who.int/intestinal_worms/strategy/en (accessed on 28 May 2019).
2. Becker, S.L.; Liwanag, H.J.; Snyder, J.S.; Akogun, O.; Belizario, V., Jr.; Freeman, M.C.; Gyorkos, T.W.; Imtiaz, R.; Keiser, J.; Krolewiecki, A.; et al. Toward the 2020 goal of soil-transmitted helminthiasis control and elimination. *PLoS Negl. Trop. Dis.* **2018**, *12*, e0006606. [CrossRef] [PubMed]

3. Fischer, K.; Gankpala, A.; Gankpala, L.; Bolay, F.K.; Curtis, K.C.; Weil, G.J.; Fischer, P.U. *Capillaria* Ova and Diagnosis of *Trichuris trichiura* Infection in Humans by Kato-Katz Smear, Liberia. *Emerg. Infect. Dis.* **2018**, *24*, 1551. [CrossRef] [PubMed]
4. Goldsmid, J.M. The African hookworm problem: An overview. In *Parasitic Helminths and Zoonoses in Africa*; Macpherson, C.N.L., Craig, P.S., Eds.; Unwin Hyman: London, UK, 1991; pp. 101–137.
5. Goldsmid, J.M. Studies on intestinal helminths in African patients at Harari Central Hospital Rhodesia. *Trans. R. Soc. Trop. Med. Hyg.* **1968**, *62*, 619–629. [CrossRef]
6. Jozefzoon, L.M.E.; Oostburg, B.F.J. Detection of hookworm and hookworm-like larvae in human fecocultures in Suriname. *Am. J. Trop. Med. Hyg.* **1994**, *51*, 501–505. [CrossRef] [PubMed]
7. Hemsrichart, V. *Ternidens deminutus* infection: First pathological report of a human case in Asia. *J. Med. Assoc. Thail.* **2005**, *88*, 1140–1143.
8. Railliet, A.; Henry, A. Le nouveau Sclérostomien (*Triodontophorus deminutus* nov. sp.) parasite de l'Homme. *C. R. Soc. Biol. Paris* **1905**, *58*, 569–571.
9. Leiper, R.T. The occurrence of a rare schlerotome of man in Nyasaland. *J. Trop. Med. Hyg.* **1908**, *2*, 1–14.
10. Brumpt, E. *Precis de Parasitologie*, 4th ed.; Masson et Cie: Paris, France, 1910.
11. Railliet, A.; Henry, A. Sur la classification des Strongylidae. II: Ankylostominae. *C. R. Soc. Bull. Paris* **1909**, *66*, 168.
12. Sandground, J.H. Studies on the life-history of *Ternidens deminutus*, a nematode parasite of man, with observations on its incidence in certain regions of Southern Africa. *Ann. Trop. Med. Parasitol.* **1931**, *25*, 147–184. [CrossRef]
13. Amberson, J.M.; Schwarz, E. *Ternidens deminutus* Railliet and Henry, a nematode parasite of man and primates. *Ann. Trop. Med. Parasitol.* **1952**, *46*, 227–237. [CrossRef]
14. Smith, A.J.; Fox, H.; White, C. Contributions to systematic helminthology. *Univ. Pa. Med. Bull.* **1908**, *20*, 283–294.
15. Sandground, J.H. *Ternidens deminutus* (Railliet & Henry) as a parasite of man in Southern Rhodesia; together with observations and experimental infection studies on an unidentified nematode parasite of man from this region. *Ann. Trop. Med. Parasitol.* **1929**, *23*, 23–31.
16. Blackie, W.K. A helminthological survey of Southern Rhodesia. *Indian Med. Gaz.* **1932**, *67*, 475.
17. Van den Berghe, L. L'existence de *Ternidens deminutus* su Katanga. *Ann. Soc. Belge Med. Trop.* **1934**, *14*, 180.
18. Webb, J.L. The helminths of the intestinal canal of man in Mauritius; and a first record of *Trichostrongylus axei* locally. *Parasitology* **1937**, *29*, 469–476. [CrossRef]
19. Metzger, S. Gastrointestinal Helminthic Parasites of Habituated Wild Chimpanzees (*Pan Troglodytes verus*) in the Taï NP, Côte d'Ivoire—Including Characterization of Cultured Helminth Developmental Stages Using Genetic Markers. Ph.D. Thesis, Freien Universität Berlin, Berlin, Germany, 2014.
20. Schindler, A.R.; De Gruijter, J.M.; Polderman, A.M.; Gasser, R.B. Definition of genetic markers in nuclear ribosomal DNA for a neglected parasite of primates, *Ternidens deminutus* (Nematoda: Strongylida)—Diagnostic and epidemiological implications. *Parasitology* **2005**, *131*, 539–546. [CrossRef]
21. Goldsmid, J.M. Ternidens infection. In *Parasitic Zoonoses*; CRC Press: Boca Raton, FL, USA, 1982; Volume II, pp. 269–288.
22. Yamaguti, S. Parasitic worms mainly from Celebes. Part 10. Nematodes of birds and mammals. *Acta Med. Okayama* **1954**, *9*, 1–19.
23. Goldsmid, J.M.; Lyons, N.F. Studies on *Ternidens deminutus* Railliet & Henry, 1909 (Nematoda) I. External morphology. *J. Helminthol.* **1973**, *47*, 119–126.
24. Goldsmid, J.M. The differentiation of *Ternidens deminutus* and hookworm ova in human infections. *Trans. R. Soc. Trop. Med. Hyg.* **1968**, *62*, 109–116. [CrossRef]
25. Goldsmid, J.M. Inorganic elements in adult *Ternidens deminutus* (Nematoda: Strongylidea: Oesophagostominae) from humans and baboons. *J. Helminthol.* **1986**, *60*, 147–148. [CrossRef]
26. Goldsmid, J.M. Studies on the life cycle and biology of *Ternidens deminutus* (Railliet & Henry, 1905), (Nematoda: Strongylidae). *J. Helminthol.* **1971**, *45*, 341–352.
27. Goldsmid, J.M. The intestinal helminthzoonoses of primates in Rhodesia. *Ann. Soc. Belge Med. Trop.* **1974**, *54*, 87–101.
28. Goldsmid, J.M. *Ternidens deminutus: A Parasitological Enigma in Rhodesia*; Faculty of Medicine Research Lecture Series No. 4; University of Rhodesia: Salisbury, Rhodesia, 1971.

29. Witenberg, G.G. Nematodiases. In *Zoonoses*; Van der Hoeden, J., Ed.; Elsevier: Amsterdam, The Netherlands, 1964; pp. 529–601.
30. Gasser, R.B.; De Gruijter, J.M.; Polderman, A.M. Insights into the epidemiology and genetic make-up of *Oesophagostomum bifurcum* from human and non-human primates using molecular tools. *Parasitology* **2006**, *132*, 453–460. [CrossRef]
31. Goldsmid, J.M. *Ternidens deminutus* (Railliet & Henry, 1909) and hookworm in Rhodesia and a review of the treatment of human infections with *T. deminutus*. *Cent. Afr. J. Med.* **1972**, *18* (Suppl. 11), 1–14.
32. Goldsmid, J.M.; Rogers, S.; Parsons, G.S.; Chambers, P.G. The intestinal protozoa and helminths infecting Africans in the Gatooma region of Rhodesia. *Cent. Afr. J. Med.* **1976**, *22*, 91–95.
33. Kilala, C.P. *Ternidens deminutus* infecting man in Southern Tanzania. *East. Afr. Med. J.* **1971**, *48*, 636–645.
34. Anthony, P.P.; McAdam, I.W.J. Helminthic pseudotumours of the bowel: Thirty-four cases of helminthoma. *Gut* **1972**, *13*, 8–16. [CrossRef]
35. Bradley, M. Rate of expulsion of *Necator americanus* and the false hookworm *Ternidens deminutus* Railliet and Henry 1909 (Nematoda) from humans following albendazole treatment. *Trans. R. Soc. Trop. Med. Hyg.* **1990**, *84*, 720. [CrossRef]
36. Bradley, M.; Chandiwana, S.K.; Bundy, D.A.P. The epidemiology and control of hookworm infection in the Burma Valley area of Zimbabwe. *Trans. R. Soc. Trop. Med. Hyg.* **1993**, *87*, 145–147. [CrossRef]
37. Guiterez, Y. *Diagnostic Pathology of Parasitic Infections with Clinical Correlations*, 2nd ed.; Oxford University Press: Oxford, UK, 2000.
38. Myers, W.M. *Pathology of Infectious Diseases: Helminthiases*; Armed Forces Institute of Pathology: Washington, DC, USA, 2000.
39. Pafčo, B.; Čížková, D.; Kreisinger, J.; Hasegawa, H.; Vallo, P.; Shutt, K.; Todd, A.; Petrželková, K.J.; Modrý, D. Metabarcoding analysis of strongylid nematode diversity in two sympatric primate species. *Sci. Rep.* **2018**, *8*, 5933. [CrossRef]
40. Bradbury, R.S.; Speare, R. Passage of *Meloidogyne* eggs in human stool: Forgotten, but not gone. *J. Clin. Microbiol.* **2015**, *53*, 1458–1459. [CrossRef]
41. Blotkamp, J.; Krepel, H.P.; Kumar, V.; Baeta, S.; Van't Noordende, J.M.; Polderman, A.M. Observations on the morphology of adults and larval stages of *Oesophagostomum* sp. isolated from man in northern Togo and Ghana. *J. Helminthol.* **1993**, *67*, 49–61. [CrossRef]
42. Goldsmid, J.M. *Ternidens deminutus* Railliet and Henry (Nematoda): A diagnostic problem in Rhodesia. *Cent. Afr. J. Med.* **1967**, *13*, 54–58.
43. Lyons, N.F.; Goldsmid, J.M. Abnormal *Ternidens deminutus* Railliet and Henry, 1909 (Nematoda) from man in Rhodesia. *J. Parasitol.* **1973**, *59*, 219–220. [CrossRef]

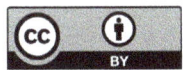

© 2019 by the author. Licensee MDPI, Basel, Switzerland. This article is an open access article distributed under the terms and conditions of the Creative Commons Attribution (CC BY) license (http://creativecommons.org/licenses/by/4.0/).

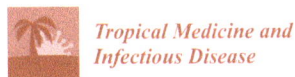

Perspective

Acute Lymphatic Filariasis Infection in United States Armed Forces Personnel Deployed to the Pacific Area of Operations during World War II Provides Important Lessons for Today

Wayne D. Melrose [1,*] and Peter A. Leggat [1,2]

1. World Health Organization Collaborating Centre for Vector-Borne and Neglected Tropical Diseases, College of Public Health, Medical and Veterinary Science, James Cook University, Townsville 4811, Australia; peter.leggat@jcu.edu.au
2. School of Public Health, Faculty of Health Sciences, University of the Witwatersrand, Johannesburg 2001, South Africa
* Correspondence: Wayne.Melrose@jcu.edu.au

Received: 19 February 2020; Accepted: 15 April 2020; Published: 17 April 2020

Abstract: The deployment of United States (US) Armed Forces personnel into the central Pacific islands of Samoa and Tonga, which is highly-endemic for lymphatic filariasis (LF), resulted in thousands of cases of the acute form of this disease and greatly reduced their ability to carry out their mission. The major driving factor for the intensity of transmission was the aggressiveness and efficiency of the *Aedes* species mosquito vectors, especially the day-biting *Ae. Polynesiensis*. The paper reminds us of the danger that tropical diseases can pose for troops sent into endemic areas and constant and careful surveillance that is required to prevent rapid resurgence of *Aedes*-transmitted LF in populations, where the LF elimination program has been successful.

Keywords: medical history; military; WW2; lymphatic filariasis; helminth; Pacific

1. Introduction

Lymphatic filariasis (LF) is a mosquito-transmitted parasitic disease caused by infection with the filarial worms, *Wuchereria bancrofti*, *Brugia malayi* and *Brugia timori*. The adult worms live within the lymphatics and the female worms liberate motile embryonic forms called microfilariae into the peripheral blood. In parts of the world where the LF vectors are *Anopheline*, *Culex* and *Mansonia* mosquitos that bite mostly at night, microfilariae numbers in the blood peak during the night (nocturnal periodicity). In the central Pacific, where the vectors are *Aedes* mosquitoes that bite mostly during the day, microfilariae numbers peak at midday (diurnal periodicity). The global burden of LF is estimated to be around 70 million and its debilitating manifestations of lymphedema, elephantiasis and hydrocele disable around 36 million making it one of the leading causes of chronic disability [1]. There is also an acute form of LF characterized by fever, lymphangitis, and lymphadenopathy and in males, scrotal inflammation [2]. This form of LF is the main focus of this paper.

In 1997, the 50th World Health Assembly passed a resolution to eliminate LF as a public health problem and, in 1999, the Pacific Program for the Elimination of LF (PacELF) was established to eliminate the disease in the 22 LF-endemic countries in the Pacific region through a strategy of annual rounds of mass drug administration (MDA) [3]. By March 2020, Cook Islands, Kiribati, Marshall Islands, Niue, Palau, Tonga, Vanuatu, Wallis and Futuna have been certified by the World Health Organization (WHO) as having achieved the elimination target and several other countries are completing the data collection required for certification and, after completing LF surveys, the Solomon Islands has been declared to be nonendemic and not requiring an MDA program [3–5]. This is an outstanding achievement, but the history of LF in the Pacific area during World War II (WW2), provides important lessons that need to be taken into account to prevent a resurgence in the disease.

2. Lymphatic Filariasis in the Pacific Region during WW2

During WW2, LF was a major health issue for the US Armed Forces stationed in filarial-endemic areas of the South Pacific and this has been comprehensively reviewed by Coggeshall [6] and Wartman [7]. Although cases occurred throughout the area, the highest number of cases occurred in the central Pacific, especially in Samoa (then consisting of "Western Samoa" and "American Samoa") and Tonga. There were 127 cases of LF reported at a field hospital in Samoa over a 4-month period [8] and in one unit stationed in Samoa, 70% of the exposed troops became infected. On Tonga-Tabu Island in Tonga, 532 men were diagnosed with LF in a single year [9].

3. The Clinical Features of LF in American Armed Forces Personnel

The very sensitive and specific filarial antigen tests that are now regarded as the "gold standard" for LF infection [1] were not available back then, but the diagnosis was not in doubt. The episodic acute attacks of malaise and fatigue, urticaria, painful inflammation and swelling of the genitalia and lymphangitis of the arms and legs, sometimes precipitated or worsened by heavy exercise, are consistent with acute LF (7,10). Surprisingly, fever was not commonly reported. Fever is commonly seen in acute LF, which is often called "filarial fever" [10], and the description of "Mumu", which is what acute LF is called in the Samoan language, stresses fever as an important symptom [6]. In 30% of all cases adult worms were removed by surgery or seen in histological sections [7] but only about 20 cases microfilaraemia were detected [7,9]. This was not surprising because microfilaraemia is very rare in acute LF. The exact reason is not known, but possible explanations are that microfilaria are trapped within inflammatory tissue, or rapidly destroyed by the acute inflammatory reaction once they enter the circulation, that the adult worms are of a single sex, or the adult females are too young to produce microfilariae [1,7,9,10]. It is also possible that low numbers of microfilaria were not detected, because of the poor sensitivity of the blood film method used at the time. Modern practice is to use more sensitive concentration techniques [1]. The most common laboratory finding was eosinophilia [7,11].

An interesting observation is that psychological disturbances were common and recorded by several authors [12–14]. Symptoms included depression, difficulty in concentrating, anxiety, insomnia and fearfulness. Some of these symptoms may have been prompted by a fear that they might develop some of the severe chronic pathology of LF such as hydrocele and elephantiasis seen in the local population, and that they would, as one writer puts it, "go home with their scrotum in a wheelbarrow" or suffer a loss of sexual function. Chronic pathology is the result of a long-standing, complex interaction between the parasite and the host's immune system, and, very importantly, the skin and tissue damaged caused by recurrent bacterial and fungal infections [1]. None of these men remained in the endemic area long enough for this to occur. The prevalence of sexual dysfunction or sterility was no higher in LF patients than in the general population [7].

4. How Long Did the Clinical Evidence of LF Persist after Returning from an Endemic Area?

No specific treatment was available for LF at that time and the length of time it took for the signs and symptoms of LF to resolve after returning from and endemic area varied. For most cases, it was 20–30 months and for others it took 3 years [7,15] and a careful evaluation of a group of cases after 15 years showed that around a third of them still suffered from acute attacks. A single case who got LF during his deployment to Samoa still complained of symptoms in 1972 [16], and one of the rare microfilaraemic cases still had microfilaria in his blood after 15 years [17,18].

5. Why Did Most of These Cases Occur in the Central Pacific Area?

The reason that Wartman and many of the other authors give, is that that the US Armed Forces personnel were in very close contact with infected local inhabitants in an area that was highly endemic for LF that was transmitted by a day-biting mosquito [7]. In addition, most of the troops' activities occurred during the day; hence their exposure rate was very high [7]. By contrast, only a small number of LF cases were recorded among the thousands of US Armed Forces personnel stationed in the Melanesian countries of Papua New Guinea, the Solomon Islands and the New Hebrides (now Vanuatu) that were also highly filarial endemic [7]. In this area, the vectors are night biting Anopheline species [1], but troops who were occupying positions and fighting both day and night would be just as exposed as their comrades in the central Pacific. In Tonga, the vectors are the mainly day-biting *Ae. tongae* and *Ae. tabu* [5]. In American Samoa and Samoa, the primary vector is the aggressive and highly efficient day-biting Ae. polynesiensis. Other vectors include Ae. samoanus (night-biting), Ae. tutuilae (night-biting), and Ae. upolensis (day-biting) [19]. *Aedes* species breed prolifically in a wide range of places such as tree holes, leaf axils, water-filled tree stumps, coconut shells and crab holes on beaches, and very importantly, in artificial containers like buckets, cans, bottles and tires, which you would expect to be present in big numbers where troops congregate. [20]. Research shows that *Ae. polynesiensis* is a more efficient LF vector than anophelines, especially when the number of circulating microfilariae is low [21]. All these factors meant that the US Armed Forces personnel on the highly-endemic islands of Samoa and Tonga, often working out in the open and wearing only minimal clothing, were constantly being attacked by large numbers of aggressive, effective and efficient LF vectors. Given these circumstances, it understandable that the number of LF cases were so high. By contrast, there are some other factors that might help explain why LF cases were lower in Melanesia, where LF and malaria are transmitted concomitantly by the same vector. It is extremely likely that the use mosquito repellent, inducing troops to cover up as much skin as possible and, later in the war, the use of Dichlorodiphenyltrichloroethane (or DDT) to combat malaria also reduced LF transmission. There is good evidence for this from the Solomon Islands where a control program against malaria resulted in elimination of LF without any specific intervention against LF.

6. So What Lessons Can Be Learned from This WW2 Experience?

Firstly, it is a very good example of how deployments can unexpectedly expose a large number of armed forces personnel to a tropical disease or other infective agent that can have a serious effect on their ability to carry out their mission. Several authors cited above point out that little was known about LF, especially its acute form, and the possible threat to the US Armed Forces personnel prior to them being sent overseas. Tropical diseases can still pose a threat to modern day military forces deployed to areas, where they are endemic, and measures must be taken to mitigate the risk [21].

Secondly, it reminds us of the importance of recognizing the acute form of LF and the need to be aware that it can occur in travelers, expatriate workers, defense force members and others who have a relatively short exposure especially where especially efficient vector mosquitoes are present [2].

Thirdly, it has very important lessons for the LF elimination program in the parts of the Pacific, where *Aedes* species are the vectors. As mentioned in the introduction, Tonga has achieved the LF elimination target [5]. Samoa and American Samoa are making progress but are struggling to meet the target with residual pockets of infection in some areas and in some populations [19]. That should be no surprise given that the main vector is *Ae. polynesiensis*. Even when the LF prevalence is brought down to the elimination target there will need to be constant vigilance against resurgence, because unlike other mosquito species, *Ae. polynesiensis* also has the ability to efficiently transmit LF when population prevalence of the parasite is low and there is a small number of circulating microfilariae [22–24]. Lack of prior exposure to LF and the lack of immune resistance undoubtedly played a part in the rapid and widespread acquisition of infection in the US Armed Forces personnel and this is acknowledged by many of the authors cited above. LF protective immunity is still poorly understood and how long it will persist in communities after elimination is achieved is not known. It must be remembered that the goal of the LF program is the elimination of LF as a public health problem. It is not an eradication program, and some active cases could still arise in the future. There is a risk that LF-infected migrants could also re-introduce the parasite, especially in places where *Aedes* is the vector [25]. Will the re-appearance of a small number of LF cases spark the sort of outbreaks in these communities that were seen in the WW2 troops, as the local population, like those US Armed Forces personnel, are now immunologically naïve towards the parasite?

Funding: This research received no external funding.

Conflicts of Interest: The authors declare no conflicts of interest.

References

1. Melrose, W.D. Lymphatic filariasis—New insights into an old disease. *Int. J. Parasitol.* **2002**, *32*, 947–960. [CrossRef]
2. Leggat, P.A.; Melrose, W.D.; Durrheim, D.N. Could it be lymphatic filariasis. *J. Travel Med.* **2004**, *11*, 56–60. [CrossRef] [PubMed]
3. World Health Organization. *Lymphatic Filariasis Fact Sheet*; WHO: Geneva, Switzerland, 2020. Available online: https://www.who.int/news-room/fact-sheets/detail/lymphatic-filariasis (accessed on 15 April 2020).
4. Carlingford, C.N.; Melrose, W.D.; Mokoia, G.; Graves, P.M.; Ichimori, K.; Capuano, C.; Kim, S.H.; Aratchige, P.; Nosa, M. Elimination of lymphatic filariasis as a public health problem in Niue under PacELF. *Trop. Med. Health* **2019**, *47*, 20. [CrossRef] [PubMed]
5. Ofanoa, R.; Ofa, T.; Padmasiri, E.A.; Kapa, D.R. Elimination of lymphatic filariasis as a public health problem from Tonga. *Trop. Med. Health* **2019**, *47*, 43. [CrossRef]
6. Coggeshall, L. Filariasis in the serviceman: Retrospect and prospect. *J. Am. Med. Assoc.* **1946**, *131*, 8–12. [CrossRef]
7. Wartman, W.B. Filariasis in American Armed Forces in World War 2. *Medicine* **1947**, *26*, 333–394. [CrossRef]
8. Engelhorn, T.D.; Wellman, W.E. Filariasis in soldiers on an island in the South Pacific. *Am. J. Med. Sci.* **1945**, *209*, 209–211.
9. Beaver, P.C. Filariasis without microfilaraemia. *Am. J. Trop. Med. Hyg.* **1970**, *19*, 181–189. [CrossRef]
10. World Health Organization. Lymphatic Filariasis. In *International Travel and Health*; WHO: Geneva, Switzerland, 2012. Available online: https://www.who.int/ith/diseases/lymphaticfilariasis/en/ (accessed on 3 April 2020).
11. King, B.G. Early filariasis diagnosis and clinical findings: Report of 268 cases in American troops. *Am. J. Trop. Med. Hyg.* **1944**, *24*, 285–288. [CrossRef]
12. Huntington, R.W.; Fogel, R.H.; Eichold, A.; Dickson, J.G. Filariasis among American Troops in a South Pacific island group. *Yale J. Biol. Med.* **1944**, *16*, 529–536.
13. Dickson, J.G.; Huntington, R.W.; Eichold, S. Filariasis in Defense Force Samoan Group. *US Navy Med. Bull.* **1943**, *41*, 1241–1251.
14. Zeligs, M.A. Psychosomatic aspects of filariasis. *J. Am. Med. Assoc.* **1945**, *128*, 1139–1142. [CrossRef]
15. Melrose, W.D.; Leggat, P.A. Lymphatic Filariasis: Disease outbreaks in military deployments from World War 2. *Mil. Med.* **2005**, *170*, 585–589. [CrossRef] [PubMed]
16. Winstead, D.K. Filariasis bancrofti and chronic illness behavior. *Mil. Med.* **1978**, *143*, 869–871. [PubMed]
17. Behm, A.W.; Hayman, J.M. The course of filariasis after removal from an endemic area. *Am. J. Med. Sci.* **1946**, *211*, 386–394. [CrossRef]
18. Trent, S.C. Reevaluation of WW2 veterans with filariasis acquired in the South Pacific. *Am. J. Trop. Med. Hyg.* **1963**, *12*, 877–887. [CrossRef] [PubMed]
19. Lau, C.L.; Sheridan, S.; Ryan, S.; Roineau, M.; Andreosso, A.; Fuimaono, S.; Tufa, J.; Graves, P.M. Detecting and confirming residual hotspots of lymphatic filariasis transmission in American Samoa 8 years after stopping mass drug administration. *PLoS Negl. Trop. Dis.* **2017**, *11*, e0005914. [CrossRef] [PubMed]
20. Burkot, T.R.; Handzel, T.; Schmaedick, M.A.; Tufa, J.; Roberts, J.M.; Graves, P.M. Productivity of natural and artificial containers for *Aedes polynesiensis* and *Aedes aegypti* in four American Samoan villages. *Med. Vet. Entomol.* **2007**, *21*, 22–29. [CrossRef] [PubMed]
21. Leggat, P.A. Tropical Diseases of Military Importance: A Centennial Perspective. *J. Mil. Vet. Health* **2010**, *18*, 25–31.
22. Southgate, B.A. The significance of low density microfilaraemia in the transmission of lymphatic filariasis parasites. *J. Trop. Med. Hyg.* **1992**, *95*, 79–86.

23. Webber, R. Eradication of *Wuchereria bancrofti* through vector control. *Trans. R. Soc. Trop. Med. Hyg.* **1979**, *76*, 722–724. [CrossRef]
24. Esterre, P.; Plichart, C.; Sechan, Y.; Nguyen, N.L. The impact of 34 years of massive DEC chemotherapy on *Wuchereria bancrofti* infection and transmission: The Maupiti cohort. *Trop. Med. Int. Health.* **2001**, *6*, 190–195. [CrossRef] [PubMed]
25. Ramaiah, K. Population migration: Implications for lymphatic filariasis elimination programmes. *PLoS Negl. Trop. Dis.* **2013**, *7*, e2079. [CrossRef] [PubMed]

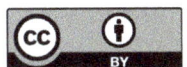

© 2020 by the authors. Licensee MDPI, Basel, Switzerland. This article is an open access article distributed under the terms and conditions of the Creative Commons Attribution (CC BY) license (http://creativecommons.org/licenses/by/4.0/).

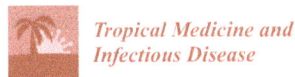

Review
A Devil of a Transmissible Cancer

Gregory M. Woods [1,*], A. Bruce Lyons [2] and Silvana S. Bettiol [2]

1. Menzies Institute for Medical Research, College of Health and Medicine, University of Tasmania, Hobart, TAS 7000, Australia
2. Tasmanian School of Medicine, College of Health and Medicine, University of Tasmania, Hobart, TAS 7000, Australia; bruce.lyons@utas.edu.au (A.B.L.); s.bettiol@utas.edu.au (S.S.B.)
* Correspondence: G.M.Woods@utas.edu.au

Received: 28 November 2019; Accepted: 27 March 2020; Published: 1 April 2020

Abstract: Devil facial tumor disease (DFTD) encompasses two independent transmissible cancers that have killed the majority of Tasmanian devils. The cancer cells are derived from Schwann cells and are spread between devils during biting, a common behavior during the mating season. The Centers for Disease Control and Prevention (CDC) defines a parasite as "An organism that lives on or in a host organism and gets its food from, or at, the expense of its host." Most cancers, including DFTD, live within a host organism and derive resources from its host, and consequently have parasitic-like features. Devil facial tumor disease is a transmissible cancer and, therefore, DFTD shares one additional feature common to most parasites. Through direct contact between devils, DFTD has spread throughout the devil population. However, unlike many parasites, the DFTD cancer cells have a simple lifecycle and do not have either independent, vector-borne, or quiescent phases. To facilitate a description of devil facial tumor disease, this review uses life cycles of parasites as an analogy.

Keywords: devil facial tumor disease; parasite; transmissible cancer; MHC; immune escape

---

For more than 50 years, Professor Goldsmid, in his memorable lectures to undergraduate students, would eloquently elaborate on the features of parasites. Some features could be attributed to cancer cells. Parasites are present in almost all species and parasitism is a hugely successful life form [1]. Cancer can be found in a variety of species [2]. Analogous to a parasite, cancer cells access various critical growth and survival resources and acquire essential nutrients from the physiology of the host [3,4]. Parasites exist within a species for most of their lifecycle and exploit the host to obtain nutrients [5]. However, in contrast to cancer, a parasite will establish a symbiotic relationship with its host by "sharing" metabolites, but not necessarily exhausting the host of its supply [5]. This review describes the life history of devil facial tumor disease (DFTD) using the analogy that DFTD can display some parasitic-like features.

Devil facial tumor disease (DFTD) was serendipitously first observed by a photographer. In 1996, Christo Baars, an amateur wildlife photographer, traveled to Tasmania, the island state of Australia, which is one of the world's most southerly islands. At 40° south, Tasmania is not a tropical island, but one where parasitic diseases have been diagnosed [6]. Christo Baars had difficulty in locating devils, but the photographs he took showed devils with grossly deformed lumps around their faces. It was possible that lesions were caused by a virus or a parasite. It was not until 2006 that results of scientific research documenting DFTD appeared in the literature [7–10]. The DFTD cancer cells displayed substantial chromosomal abnormalities. Remarkably, all DFTD cancer cells shared the same multiple chromosome abnormalities. As the karyotypes were too consistent to be considered coincidental, it led to the now accepted hypothesis that DFTD is an infectious cancer, rather than caused by a virus or parasite [10].

In 2014, a second, and independent, transmissible cancer was detected in south-east Tasmania [11]. Consequently, DFTD comprises two independent transmissible cancers, DFT1 (first identified in 1996) and DFT2 (first identified in 2014). DFT2 is currently restricted to a small pocket in the southeast of the island, whereas DFT1 has been transmitted across most of mainland Tasmania. Throughout this review, DFTD will refer to both DFT1 and DFT2; DFT1 will refer to the devil facial tumor disease first observed in 2006 and DFT2 will refer to the devil facial tumor disease first observed in 2014.

The infectious nature of the DFTD cancer cells is consistent with an infectious parasitic disease, but the parasite is a cancer cell, not an infectious microorganism. DFTD cancer cells are transmitted to another Tasmanian devil, re-establishing cancer, and then the transmission process is repeated. The DFTD cancer cells could be considered analogous to a parasite as they share other features. The suggestion that DFTD is a parasitic disease was proposed at a free public event in 2012 hosted by the Australian Society for Parasitology and Inspiring Australia [12]). Ujvari and colleagues suggested that "DFTD should be considered an evolving parasite that, like parasites, can alter life-history traits" [13,14]. For DFTD to be considered a parasite, specific criteria must be satisfied. The Centers for Disease Control and Prevention (CDC) defined a parasite as "An organism that lives on or in a host organism and gets its food from or at the expense of its host." [15]. From this simple definition, DFTD and some parasites share similar features.

DFTD cancer cells (DFT1 and DFT2) establish a cancer mass in the oral and/or facial regions, causing gross facial deformities (Figure 1A,B). Leishmania can cause a parasitic infection that produces a facial disfigurement. However, the facial disfigurement caused by Leishmania is usually a result of inflammation, whereas the facial disfigurement associated with DFTD is a combination of the cancer mass and inflammatory response, including ulceration (as shown in Figure 1).

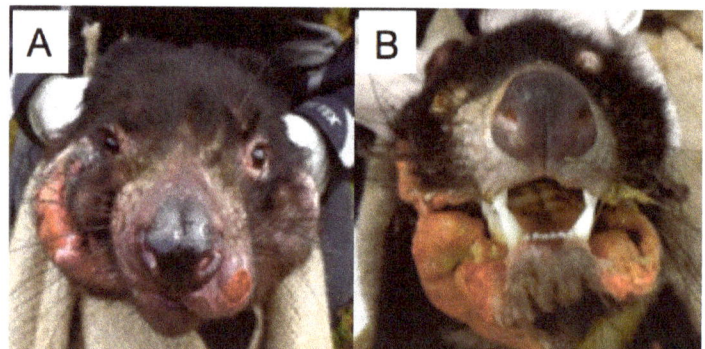

Figure 1. Gross facial deformities caused by (**A**) devil facial tumor disease 1 (DFT1) and (**B**) DFT2.

Concerning transmission, DFTD cancer cells benefit from the aggressive behavior of Tasmanian devils, a common occurrence during the mating season. Many parasites can be directly transmitted from diseased hosts to healthy recipients, also during the mating season. However, it is often the act of coitus, rather than biting, that allows direct parasite transmission [16]. With Tasmanian devils, however, it is biting that facilitates cancer cell transmission. The biting behavior of devils can be an aggressive ritual, with many of the bites occurring on the face [17]. These bites can cause penetrating wounds, ideal for inoculation. Ironically, the most reproductively "fit" devils are those more likely to become infected [18]. In contrast, diseases caused by parasites such as *Cryptosporidium* are linked to the immune status of the host. Although exposure may not discriminate, cryptosporidiosis primarily affects immunocompromised hosts [19]. The biting injuries that devils receive suggest that the dominant (fit) individuals are mostly responsible for transmission. Dominant devils have a higher incidence of DFT1 than submissive devils. Consequently, as the initial tumors are more likely to be inside the oral cavity, it is feasible that the dominant individuals are biting into the tumors of diseased devils [20]. The dominant and now diseased devils could then transmit DFTD when they bite a submissive devil on the face, thereby establishing a continuous mode of transmission. A mode of transmission is an essential prerequisite for any parasite. Devil biting occurs among males, among females, and between males and females. It is mostly the adult devils, but occasionally the sub-adult devils, that are aggressive. Via biting, DFTD is rapidly spread throughout the mature male and female devil population. Similarly, rabies is transmitted through biting [21]. In contrast, parasite transmission through biting usually requires an intermediate vector. Examples in humans include the anopheles mosquitoes transmitting malaria [22] and sandflies transmitting leishmaniasis [23].

Within ten years following the first observation, DFT1 spread from one devil to 51% of the Tasmanian devil population [7]. Within 20 years, the devil population had declined by approximately 80% [24]. Some devil populations lost 95% of their individuals [24,25]. During this time, it appeared that all devils with DFTD would die within 12 months [26]. This is contrary to many parasitic diseases where the parasite does not always kill its host and could be considered as "cohabitants" [27]. However, devils with DFT1 survive long enough to allow the transmission of some cancer cells to a healthy host, allowing perpetuation of the DFT1 cancer cell lineage. With limited evidence of resistance to DFT1 and the disease sweeping through the devil population, early estimates predicted that extinction could occur within 25–35 years since the first recorded case [25].

Extinction is not an ideal situation for any parasite as loss of the parasite's sole host would correlate to extinction of the parasite. Evidence has been gradually accumulating that some Tasmanian devils can show an immune response to DFTD. Signs of recovery from DFT1, with an associated immune response, were reported in four devils [28], indicating that although recovery from DFT1 is a rare event, it does occur. By comparing DNA from Tasmanian devils collected before DFT1 arrival with DNA collected from devils collected after DFT1 arrival, Epstein and colleagues proposed that devils are rapidly evolving in response to DFT1 [29]. Evidence for recovery from DFT1 combined with the proposal of rapid evolution of devils to DFT1 provides hope for the long-term persistence of Tasmanian devils. This latter point has been proposed following mathematical modeling of devil populations, up to ten years following DFT1 emergence. The simulation modeling predicted a 21% possibility of devil extinction within 100 years following DFT1. There was a 22% chance of devils living with DFT1 and a 57% chance that DFT1 would disappear [30]. However, this study was only based on DFT1 and did not consider the impact of the second cancer, DFT2. The key message is that current evidence does not support extinction of the Tasmanian devil, thus providing "security" for the long-term presence of DFTD (DFT1 and/or DFT2). Consequently, the parasitic-existence of DFTD and co-evolution with Tasmanian devils will be maintained for the next 100 years. Long-term existence is a critical pre-requisite for any parasite. It is possible that, when a parasite first infected a species, death occurred in almost 100% of the hosts. Gradually, evolution of the host and parasite occurred, allowing the host and parasite to co-exist in equilibrium. It is possible that we are witnessing the early stages of co-evolution of Tasmanian devils and DFTD.

For DFTD to be analogous to a parasite, it would have to be the DFTD cancer cells that are transmitted, rather than a virus (e.g., papillomavirus), that independently induced cancer. The transmitted DFTD cancer cells would establish a cancer in the new host. If this were the case, the cancer cells in the new host devil would be identical to the DFTD cancer cells in the original host devil. As discussed above, the consistency of the chromosomal changes meant that it would be too much of a coincidence for the DFT1 cancer cells to share similar complex chromosomal rearrangements if DFT1 had arisen independently in every diseased devil [31–33]. Other studies that support that the DFT1 cancer cells are the etiological agents and thus transmitted between devils include microsatellite and major histocompatibility complex class I (MHC-I) genotyping of host and DFTD cancer cells [34,35]. The potential discovery of a second transmissible cancer, DFT2, provoked an immediate analysis. A thorough examination confirmed the cancer cells to be the aetiological agent and, therefore, DFT2 was a second transmissible cancer [11,36]. The conclusion from all the molecular and genetic studies of DFT1 and DFT2 is that host tissue DNA and cancer cell DNA are different. The DFTD cancers could not have arisen from any host tissue. Such a situation with the DFTD cancer cells is analogous to the transmission of parasitic diseases, as a parasite is not derived from host tissue.

Once DFTD cancer cells or parasites are transmitted to a new host, the cells are confronted with an almost impenetrable barrier. The host's immune response is a major reason that transmissible cancers are extremely rare. In contrast, parasite transmission is far from rare, as parasites have developed strategies to subvert the host's immune system (Table 1). For DFTD cancer cells to avoid recognition by the host's immune system, some of the strategies outlined in Table 1 need to be adopted. Although it is possible for the devil's immune system to produce an immune response to DFTD cells [37], wild devils with DFTD rarely produce an immune response against the transmitted cancer cells [38]. This is despite Tasmanian devils having a competent immune system [39–41]. Consequently, the DFTD cancer cells must have developed effective immune escape mechanisms.

Table 1. A range of immune escape strategies utilized by parasites.

Immune Escape Strategies	Parasite Example
Avoid immune recognition	*Plasmodium* spp
Quiescence	*Plasmodium* spp
Avoid phagocytosis	*Toxoplasma gondii*
Suppress the host's immune response	*Trichinella spiralis*
Block natural killer (NK) cells	*Plasmodium falciparum*
Interfere with antigen processing	*Plasmodium* spp
Modify antigen surface identity	*Giardia Lamblia*

Adapted from [42].

A perusal of Table 1 provides potential mechanisms employed by parasites that DFTD cancer cells could also use to avoid the host's immune response. Investigations into the immune system of the Tasmanian devil have not identified immune deficiencies that could explain how DFTD cells can be transmitted without inducing an immune response. Within the limitations of reagent availability, a consequence of working with a unique species, assessment of lymphoid architecture, and cellular and humoral immune responses revealed a competent immune system [39–41,43]. The toll-like receptors of devil innate immune cells are functional, allowing recognition and reaction to a range of pathogens, providing evidence for a competent innate immune system [44]. Immunized devils can produce an immune response to DFTD cells [37,45], activated lymphocytes can kill DFTD cells, and skin grafts are rejected [46]. Therefore, deficiencies in allorecognition mechanisms and anti-tumor immunity do not explain why the transmitted DFTD cancer cells establish in the recipient devil. Immunocompromised hosts are susceptible to some parasitic infections, such as *Cryptosporidium* [47,48]. Furthermore, and unlike helminth parasites [49], it is unlikely that DFTD cancer cells suppress the host's immune system in order to establish. This is because Tasmanian devils with DFT1 appear to have an immune system comparable to healthy devils [39]. DFTD cancer cells do not behave like the helminth parasites by suppressing the immune system, or like *Cryptosporidium* by affecting immunosuppressed hosts. The DFTD cancer cells, similar to parasites, must have developed mechanisms to escape the host's immune response. However, DFTD cancer cells have developed different immune escape mechanisms to parasites.

The vast majority of devils with DFTD do not show evidence for an immune response to the DFTD cancer cells. The most likely immune escape mechanism would be the capacity of the DFTD cancer cells to avoid immune recognition. The DFTD (DFT1 and DFT2) cancer cells are eukaryotic, derived from devil tissue, and Schwann cell in origin [50,51]. Therefore, they do not need to employ sophisticated immune avoidance strategies. DFTD cells only need to avoid allogeneic immune recognition. Eukaryotic cells express molecules of the major histocompatibility complex (MHC). There are two classes; MHC class I (MHC-I) and MHC class II (MHC-II). The relevance of MHC-I and MHC-II is that they represent the final step of antigen processing and present antigen peptide to T cells.

Avoidance of antigen processing and antigen presentation to T cells provides an effective escape mechanism. Some parasitic protozoa can cleverly manipulate antigen presentation to avoid inducing an immune response [52]. To circumvent antigen processing and presentation and avoid immune recognition, DFT1 cancer cells employ a simple strategy; DFT1 cancer cells do not express MHC molecules [53]. Epigenetic downregulation of critical MHC processing genes prevents the MHC molecules from being expressed on the surface of the DFT1 cancer cells. As no DFT1 antigens are presented to T cells, the DFT1 cancer cells are effectively "invisible" to the host's immune system. Although the absence of MHC expression is a simple strategy, a similarity to some parasites is that the mechanisms accounting for MHC-I downregulation are complex. Histone deacetylase appears to epigenetically silence genes such as β_2m, TAP1, and TAP2, thereby preventing MHC-I expression on the DFTD cancer cells. As the antigen processing genes are present, but downregulated, their expression can be restored following exposure to trichostatin A (TSA) or interferon-γ (IFN-γ) [53]. Further analysis of the antigen processing pathway revealed that the ERBB–STAT3 axis was activated in DFT1 cancer cells [54]. The activated genes in the ERBB–STAT3 axis had two effects: the promotion of cell growth and the downregulation of MHC-I. The complexity of MHC-I downregulation was exemplified following a genome-wide clustered regularly interspaced short palindromic repeats (CRISPR)-CRISPR-associated protein (Cas)9 (CRISPR/Cas9) screen of DFT1 cancer cells. The epigenetic silencing of the MHC-I processing pathway in DFT1 was also related to the polycomb repressive complex-2 (PRC2) [55].

Upregulation of MHC-I expression on the DFTD cancer cells has provided a useful strategy towards a vaccine or immunotherapy [56,57]. Similar to many parasitic diseases, such as malaria [58], producing an effective vaccine has proved elusive. The first phase 3 clinical trial of a malaria vaccine was partially effective as it prevented approximately 40% of malaria cases in children during the four-year follow-up [59]. A prototype vaccine using killed DFTD cancer cells has only been partially effective (Pye, R; personal communication). The pathway to an effective vaccine to protect against DFTD may require strategies that have been attempted with parasites such as isolating T cell epitopes for malaria [60] or a combination with drugs that interfere with the ERBB–STAT3 axis [54].

Theoretically, the absence of MHC-I expression on the membrane of DFTD cancer cells would make the cells targets for natural killer (NK) cells. Despite genetic and immunohistochemical evidence for the presence of NK cells [61,62], there is no verification for spontaneous NK cell responses to DFTD cancer cells [61]. Mitogen-activated peripheral blood lymphocytes can kill DFTD cancer cells. Therefore, NK cell activation appears to be prevented by the DFT1 cancer cells. A strategy used by *Plasmodium falciparum* is that, following infection of red blood cells, the *Plasmodium falciparum* produces inhibitory receptors that are expressed on the infected red blood cells [63]. These inhibitory receptors, collectively known as a repetitive interspersed family (RIFIN), bind to B cells and NK cells, and prevent activation, thereby preventing NK cell activation and protection of the parasite. It is unknown why DFTD cancer cells fail to activate NK cells, but they may express inhibitory molecules, and thus utilize a similar strategy to *Plasmodium falciparum*. The cancer cells of the second transmissible cancer, DFT2, express non-classical MHC molecules [64], which are known to inhibit T cell and NK cell function.

The above provides support for classifying the DFTD cancer cells as parasites, but one key element is missing. Parasites usually have a complex life cycle that can involve more than one host. The life cycle of Leishmania involves humans and sand flies, and the formation of amastigotes and promastigotes. *Toxoplasma gondii* infects humans and cats, and the life cycle involves tachyzoites, bradyzoites, sporozoites, trophozoites, merozoites, and oocytes. The *Toxoplasma* oocysts have a free-living phase as they can survive in cat feces in the environment. In contrast, DFTD cancer cells have a simple life cycle (basically cell division) with no quiescent phase and no free-living stage. Transmission of DFTD occurs directly between devils and the cancer cells will not survive in the environment. It is unlikely that DFTD can infect any other species. Marsupials that coexist with devils have never shown signs of DFTD. Furthermore, mice injected with viable DFTD cancer cells readily reject the foreign cancer cells [65].

As parasites exist within everchanging and hostile environments, natural selection shapes how parasites adapt and survive [66]. Cancer cells also live within a changing environment and need to compete for the host's resources. Similar to parasites, cancer cells driven by genetic and epigenetic changes are continually evolving [67]. Cancer as an ongoing evolutionary process has been suggested [68]. Random genetic or epigenetic events may confer a selective advantage and drive evolutionary processes [69]. Parasitic diseases and cancer both display evolutionary traits. To detect evidence of evolution, Ujvari and colleagues investigated the methylation patterns of DFTD cells from a range of cancers that were separated by time [14]. The authors discovered complex changes in methylation patterns with DFTD. However, demethylation increased over time and this correlated with an increase in the genes for the DNA-demethylase enzymes MBD2 and MB4. The conclusion that "DFTD should not be treated as a static entity, but rather as an evolving parasite with epigenetic plasticity" [14], is one of the earliest considerations of DFTD as a parasite.

Ujvari and colleagues extended the theme that cancer and parasites have similarities. They compared the life-history traits (e.g., fecundity, survival) of parasites and cancers (including DFTD) and showed that cancers and parasites had similar effects on life history [13]. Specifically, they noted the effect of DFTD on fecundity, which increased the proportion of devils displaying precocious sexual maturity and early reproduction [70]. Cancer cells and parasites share the exploitation of the host for resources, resulting in diminishing health. It is known that a consequence of parasites exploiting host resources is an evolution of life-history traits, including reproduction and lifespan. As mentioned above, DFTD appears to have a similar effect on life-history traits. Using DFTD as a model cancer, Russell and colleagues concluded that parasites and DFTD can affect devil life-history traits [71]. The canine transmissible venereal tumor (CTVT) has been referred to as a "parasitic tumor" [72]. Another approach to comparing parasites to cancer was performed by Lun and colleagues [73]. The authors highlighted that cancer could occur in many species, including *Toxoplasma gondii*. The protozoan cancer has the potential to cause death in mammals. Parallels were identified between protozoan parasites and cancer cells. Devil facial tumor disease was used as an example of a transmissible cancer that existed as an autonomous organism and could be considered an "asexually duplicating unicellular pathogen" [73].

At the free public event in 2012, Parasite Encounters in the Wild [12], the audience was asked: "Is DFTD the perfect parasite?". The unanimous response was "No". While it is clear that DFTD is not a parasite, by comparing DFTD to a parasitic disease, similar features are revealed. Such a comparison may facilitate an understanding of the life cycle and mode of transmission of this unique and fascinating cancer.

Author Contributions: Conceptualization, G.M.W., A.B.L. and S.S.B.; methodology, G.M.W., A.B.L. and S.S.B.; validation, G.M.W., A.B.L. and S.S.B.; formal analysis, G.M.W.; investigation, G.M.W.; resources, G.M.W. and A.B.L.; data curation, G.M.W. and A.B.L.; writing—original draft preparation, G.M.W.; writing—review and editing, G.M.W., A.B.L. and S.S.B.; funding acquisition, G.M.W. and A.B.L. All authors have read and agreed to the published version of the manuscript.

Funding: This research was supported by the Australian Research Council (DP130100715 and DP180100520), Wildcare-Saffire Devil Fund, and the University of Tasmania Foundation through funds raised by the Save the Tasmanian Devil Appeal.

Acknowledgments: The authors thank Camila Espejo for providing the image for Figure 1A, and Ruth Pye, Liz Pulo, and Sarah Peck for providing the image for Figure 1B.

Conflicts of Interest: The authors declare no conflict of interest.

References

1. Poulin, R.; Morand, S. The Diversity of Parasites. *Q. Rev. Biol.* **2000**, *75*, 277–293. [CrossRef]
2. Aktipis, C.A.; Boddy, A.M.; Jansen, G.; Hibner, U.; Hochberg, M.E.; Maley, C.C.; Wilkinson, G.S. Cancer across the tree of life: Cooperation and cheating in multicellularity. *Philos. Trans. R. Soc. Lond. Ser. B Biol. Sci.* **2015**, *370*. [CrossRef]
3. Icard, P.; Lincet, H. [The cancer tumor: A metabolic parasite?]. *Bull. Cancer* **2013**, *100*, 427–433. [CrossRef] [PubMed]

4. Pavlova, N.N.; Thompson, C.B. The Emerging Hallmarks of Cancer Metabolism. *Cell Metab.* **2016**, *23*, 27–47. [CrossRef] [PubMed]
5. Zuzarte-Luis, V.; Mota, M.M. Parasite Sensing of Host Nutrients and Environmental Cues. *Cell Host Microbe* **2018**, *23*, 749–758. [CrossRef] [PubMed]
6. Goldsmid, J.M.; Bettiol, S.S. Global Medicine, Parasites, and Tasmania. *Trop. Med. Infect. Dis.* **2020**, *5*, 7. [CrossRef]
7. Hawkins, C.E.; Baars, C.; Hesterman, H.; Hocking, G.J.; Jones, M.E.; Lazenby, B.; Mann, D.; Mooney, N.; Pemberton, D.; Pyecroft, S.; et al. Emerging disease and population decline of an island endemic, the Tasmanian devil *Sarcophilus harrisii*. *Biol. Conserv.* **2006**, *131*, 307–324. [CrossRef]
8. Loh, R.; Bergfeld, J.; Hayes, D.; O'Hara, A.; Pyecroft, S.; Raidal, S.; Sharpe, R. The pathology of devil facial tumor disease (DFTD) in Tasmanian devils (*Sarcophilus harrisii*). *Vet. Pathol.* **2006**, *43*, 890–895. [CrossRef] [PubMed]
9. Loh, R.; Hayes, D.; Mahjoor, A.; O'Hara, A.; Pyecroft, S.; Raidal, S. The immunohistochemical characterization of devil facial tumor disease (DFTD) in the Tasmanian Devil (*Sarcophilus harrisii*). *Vet. Pathol.* **2006**, *43*, 896–903. [CrossRef] [PubMed]
10. Pearse, A.M.; Swift, K. Allograft theory: Transmission of devil facial-tumor disease. *Nature* **2006**, *439*, 549. [CrossRef] [PubMed]
11. Pye, R.J.; Pemberton, D.; Tovar, C.; Tubio, J.M.; Dun, K.A.; Fox, S.; Darby, J.; Hayes, D.; Knowles, G.W.; Kreiss, A.; et al. A second transmissible cancer in Tasmanian devils. *Proc. Natl. Acad. Sci. USA* **2016**, *113*, 374–378. [CrossRef] [PubMed]
12. Woods, G.M.; Thompson, R.; Beveridge, I.; Kelly, A. Parasite Encounters in the Wild. Available online: https://www.parasite.org.au/outreach/inspiring-australia/ (accessed on 20 November 2019).
13. Ujvari, B.; Beckmann, C.; Biro, P.A.; Arnal, A.; Tasiemski, A.; Massol, F.; Salzet, M.; Mery, F.; Boidin-Wichlacz, C.; Misse, D.; et al. Cancer and life-history traits: Lessons from host-parasite interactions. *Parasitology* **2016**, *143*, 533–541. [CrossRef]
14. Ujvari, B.; Pearse, A.M.; Peck, S.; Harmsen, C.; Taylor, R.; Pyecroft, S.; Madsen, T.; Papenfuss, A.T.; Belov, K. Evolution of a contagious cancer: Epigenetic variation in devil facial tumor disease. *Proc. Biol. Sci.* **2013**, *280*. [CrossRef] [PubMed]
15. Centers for Disease Control and Prevention. About Parasites. Available online: https://www.cdc.gov/parasites/about.html (accessed on 19 November 2019).
16. Gardai, S.J.; McPhillips, K.A.; Frasch, S.C.; Janssen, W.J.; Starefeldt, A.; Murphy-Ullrich, J.E.; Bratton, D.L.; Oldenborg, P.A.; Michalak, M.; Henson, P.M. Cell-surface calreticulin initiates clearance of viable or apoptotic cells through trans-activation of LRP on the phagocyte. *Cell* **2005**, *123*, 321–334. [CrossRef] [PubMed]
17. Hamede, R.K.; McCallum, H.; Jones, M.E. Seasonal, demographic and density-related patterns of contact between Tasmanian devils (*Sarcophilus harrisii*): Implications for transmission of devil facial tumor disease. *Austral Ecol.* **2008**, *33*, 614–622. [CrossRef]
18. Wells, K.; Hamede, R.K.; Kerlin, D.H.; Storfer, A.; Hohenlohe, P.A.; Jones, M.E.; McCallum, H.I. Infection of the fittest: Devil facial tumor disease has greatest effect on individuals with highest reproductive output. *Ecol. Lett.* **2017**, *20*, 770–778. [CrossRef]
19. Laurent, F.; Lacroix-Lamande, S. Innate immune responses play a key role in controlling infection of the intestinal epithelium by *Cryptosporidium*. *Int. J. Parasitol.* **2017**, *47*, 711–721. [CrossRef]
20. Hamede, R.K.; McCallum, H.; Jones, M. Biting injuries and transmission of Tasmanian devil facial tumor disease. *J. Anim. Ecol.* **2013**, *82*, 182–190. [CrossRef]
21. Fooks, A.R.; Banyard, A.C.; Horton, D.L.; Johnson, N.; McElhinney, L.M.; Jackson, A.C. Current status of rabies and prospects for elimination. *Lancet* **2014**, *384*, 1389–1399. [CrossRef]
22. Meibalan, E.; Marti, M. Biology of Malaria Transmission. *Cold Spring Harb. Perspect. Med.* **2017**, *7*. [CrossRef]
23. Bates, P.A. Transmission of Leishmania metacyclic promastigotes by phlebotomine sand flies. *Int. J. Parasitol.* **2007**, *37*, 1097–1106. [CrossRef] [PubMed]
24. Lazenby, B.T.; Tobler, M.W.; Brown, W.E.; Hawkins, C.E.; Hocking, G.J.; Hume, F.; Huxtable, S.; Iles, P.; Jones, M.E.; Lawrence, C.; et al. Density trends and demographic signals uncover the long-term impact of transmissible cancer in Tasmanian devils. *J. Appl. Ecol.* **2018**, *55*, 1368–1379. [CrossRef] [PubMed]

25. McCallum, H.; Tompkins, D.M.; Jones, M.; Lachish, S.; Marvanek, S.; Lazenby, B.; Hocking, G.; Wiersma, J.; Hawkins, C.E. Distribution and impacts of Tasmanian devil facial tumor disease. *Ecohealth* **2007**, *4*, 318–325. [CrossRef]
26. Hamede, R.K.; Lachish, S.; Belov, K.; Woods, G.; Kreiss, A.; Pearse, A.M.; Lazenby, B.; Jones, M.; McCallum, H. Reduced effect of Tasmanian devil facial tumor disease at the disease front. *Conserv. Biol.* **2012**, *26*, 124–134. [CrossRef] [PubMed]
27. Vannier-Santos, M.A.; Lenzi, H.L. Parasites or cohabitants: Cruel omnipresent usurpers or creative "eminences grises"? *J. Parasitol. Res.* **2011**, *2011*. [CrossRef] [PubMed]
28. Pye, R.J.; Hamede, R.; Siddle, H.V.; Caldwell, A.; Knowles, G.W.; Swift, K.; Kreiss, A.; Jones, M.E.; Lyons, A.B.; Woods, G.M. Demonstration of immune responses against devil facial tumor disease in wild Tasmanian devils. *Biol. Lett.* **2016**, *12*. [CrossRef]
29. Epstein, B.; Jones, M.; Hamede, R.; Hendricks, S.; McCallum, H.; Murchison, E.P.; Schonfeld, B.; Wiench, C.; Hohenlohe, P.; Storfer, A. Rapid evolutionary response to a transmissible cancer in Tasmanian devils. *Nat. Commun.* **2016**, *7*. [CrossRef]
30. Wells, K.; Hamede, R.K.; Jones, M.E.; Hohenlohe, P.A.; Storfer, A.; McCallum, H.I. Individual and temporal variation in pathogen load predicts long-term impacts of an emerging infectious disease. *Ecology* **2019**, *100*, e02613. [CrossRef]
31. Deakin, J.E.; Papenfuss, A.T.; Belov, K.; Cross, J.G.; Coggill, P.; Palmer, S.; Sims, S.; Speed, T.P.; Beck, S.; Graves, J.A. Evolution and comparative analysis of the MHC Class III inflammatory region. *BMC Genom.* **2006**, *7*, 281. [CrossRef]
32. Deakin, J.E.; Bender, H.S.; Pearse, A.M.; Rens, W.; O'Brien, P.C.; Ferguson-Smith, M.A.; Cheng, Y.; Morris, K.; Taylor, R.; Stuart, A.; et al. Genomic restructuring in the Tasmanian devil facial tumor: Chromosome painting and gene mapping provide clues to evolution of a transmissible tumor. *PLoS Genet.* **2012**, *8*, e1002483. [CrossRef]
33. Murchison, E.P.; Schulz-Trieglaff, O.B.; Ning, Z.; Alexandrov, L.B.; Bauer, M.J.; Fu, B.; Hims, M.; Ding, Z.; Ivakhno, S.; Stewart, C.; et al. Genome sequencing and analysis of the Tasmanian devil and its transmissible cancer. *Cell* **2012**, *148*, 780–791. [CrossRef] [PubMed]
34. Siddle, H.V.; Kreiss, A.; Eldridge, M.D.; Noonan, E.; Clarke, C.J.; Pycroft, S.; Woods, G.M.; Belov, K. Transmission of a fatal clonal tumor by biting occurs due to depleted MHC diversity in a threatened carnivorous marsupial. *Proc. Natl. Acad. Sci. USA* **2007**, *104*, 16221–16226. [CrossRef] [PubMed]
35. Miller, W.; Hayes, V.M.; Ratan, A.; Petersen, D.C.; Wittekindt, N.E.; Miller, J.; Walenz, B.; Knight, J.; Qi, J.; Zhao, F.; et al. Genetic diversity and population structure of the endangered marsupial *Sarcophilus harrisii* (Tasmanian devil). *Proc. Natl. Acad. Sci. USA* **2011**, *108*, 12348–12353. [CrossRef] [PubMed]
36. Stammnitz, M.R.; Coorens, T.H.H.; Gori, K.C.; Hayes, D.; Fu, B.; Wang, J.; Martin-Herranz, D.E.; Alexandrov, L.B.; Baez-Ortega, A.; Barthorpe, S.; et al. The origins and vulnerabilities of two transmissible cancers in Tasmanian devils. *Cancer Cell* **2018**, *33*, 607–619.e615. [CrossRef] [PubMed]
37. Kreiss, A.; Brown, G.K.; Tovar, C.; Lyons, A.B.; Woods, G.M. Evidence for induction of humoral and cytotoxic immune responses against devil facial tumor disease cells in Tasmanian devils (*Sarcophilus harrisii*) immunized with killed cell preparations. *Vaccine* **2015**, *33*, 3016–3025. [CrossRef]
38. Woods, G.M.; Kreiss, A.; Belov, K.; Siddle, H.V.; Obendorf, D.L.; Muller, H.K. The immune response of the Tasmanian Devil (*Sarcophilus harrisii*) and devil facial tumor disease. *Ecohealth* **2007**, *4*, 338–345. [CrossRef]
39. Kreiss, A.; Fox, N.; Bergfeld, J.; Quinn, S.J.; Pycroft, S.; Woods, G.M. Assessment of cellular immune responses of healthy and diseased Tasmanian devils (*Sarcophilus harrisii*). *Dev. Comp. Immunol.* **2008**, *32*, 544–553. [CrossRef]
40. Kreiss, A.; Wells, B.; Woods, G.M. The humoral immune response of the Tasmanian devil (*Sarcophilus harrisii*) against horse red blood cells. *Vet. Immunol. Immunopathol.* **2009**, *130*, 135–137. [CrossRef]
41. Kreiss, A.; Obendorf, D.L.; Hemsley, S.; Canfield, P.J.; Woods, G.M. A histological and immunohistochemical analysis of lymphoid tissues of the Tasmanian devil. *Anat. Rec.* **2009**, *292*, 611–620. [CrossRef]
42. Schmid-Hempel, P. Parasite immune evasion: A momentous molecular war. *Trends Ecol. Evol.* **2008**, *23*, 318–326. [CrossRef]

43. Howson, L.J.; Morris, K.M.; Kobayashi, T.; Tovar, C.; Kreiss, A.; Papenfuss, A.T.; Corcoran, L.; Belov, K.; Woods, G.M. Identification of dendritic cells, B cell and T cell subsets in Tasmanian devil lymphoid tissue; evidence for poor immune cell infiltration into devil facial tumors. *Anat. Rec.* **2014**, *297*, 925–938. [CrossRef] [PubMed]
44. Patchett, A.L.; Latham, R.; Brettingham-Moore, K.H.; Tovar, C.; Lyons, A.B.; Woods, G.M. Toll-like receptor signaling is functional in immune cells of the endangered Tasmanian devil. *Dev. Comp. Immunol.* **2015**, *53*, 123–133. [CrossRef] [PubMed]
45. Brown, G.K.; Tovar, C.; Cooray, A.A.; Kreiss, A.; Darby, J.; Murphy, J.M.; Corcoran, L.M.; Bettiol, S.S.; Lyons, A.B.; Woods, G.M. Mitogen activated Tasmanian devil blood mononuclear cells kill devil facial tumor disease cells. *Immunol. Cell Biol.* **2016**, *94*, 673–679. [CrossRef]
46. Kreiss, A.; Cheng, Y.; Kimble, F.; Wells, B.; Donovan, S.; Belov, K.; Woods, G.M. Allorecognition in the Tasmanian devil (*Sarcophilus harrisii*), an endangered marsupial species with limited genetic diversity. *PLoS ONE* **2011**, *6*, e22402. [CrossRef] [PubMed]
47. Marcos, L.A.; Gotuzzo, E. Intestinal protozoan infections in the immunocompromised host. *Curr. Opin. Infect. Dis.* **2013**, *26*, 295–301. [CrossRef] [PubMed]
48. Siddiqui, Z.A. An overview of parasitic infections of the gastro-intestinal tract in developed countries affecting immunocompromised individuals. *J. Parasit. Dis.* **2017**, *41*, 621–626. [CrossRef]
49. Maizels, R.M.; McSorley, H.J. Regulation of the host immune system by helminth parasites. *J. Allergy Clin. Immunol.* **2016**, *138*, 666–675. [CrossRef]
50. Patchett, A.L.; Coorens, T.H.H.; Darby, J.; Wilson, R.; McKay, M.J.; Kamath, K.S.; Rubin, A.; Wakefield, M.; McIntosh, L.; Mangiola, S.; et al. Two of a kind: Transmissible Schwann cell cancers in the endangered Tasmanian devil (*Sarcophilus harrisii*). *Cell. Mol. Life Sci.* **2019**. [CrossRef]
51. Murchison, E.P.; Tovar, C.; Hsu, A.; Bender, H.S.; Kheradpour, P.; Rebbeck, C.A.; Obendorf, D.; Conlan, C.; Bahlo, M.; Blizzard, C.A.; et al. The Tasmanian devil transcriptome reveals Schwann cell origins of a clonally transmissible cancer. *Science* **2010**, *327*, 84–87. [CrossRef]
52. Sacks, D.; Sher, A. Evasion of innate immunity by parasitic protozoa. *Nat. Immunol.* **2002**, *3*, 1041–1047. [CrossRef] [PubMed]
53. Siddle, H.V.; Kreiss, A.; Tovar, C.; Yuen, C.K.; Cheng, Y.Y.; Belov, K.; Swift, K.; Pearse, A.M.; Hamede, R.; Jones, M.E.; et al. Reversible epigenetic down-regulation of MHC molecules by devil facial tumor disease illustrates immune escape by a contagious cancer. *Proc. Natl. Acad. Sci. USA* **2013**, *110*, 5103–5108. [CrossRef] [PubMed]
54. Kosack, L.; Wingelhofer, B.; Popa, A.; Orlova, A.; Agerer, B.; Vilagos, B.; Majek, P.; Parapatics, K.; Lercher, A.; Ringler, A.; et al. The ERBB-STAT3 Axis Drives Tasmanian Devil Facial Tumor Disease. *Cancer Cell* **2019**, *35*. [CrossRef] [PubMed]
55. Burr, M.L.; Sparbier, C.E.; Chan, K.L.; Chan, Y.C.; Kersbergen, A.; Lam, E.Y.N.; Azidis-Yates, E.; Vassiliadis, D.; Bell, C.C.; Gilan, O.; et al. An Evolutionarily Conserved Function of Polycomb Silences the MHC Class I Antigen Presentation Pathway and Enables Immune Evasion in Cancer. *Cancer Cell* **2019**, *36*. [CrossRef] [PubMed]
56. Tovar, C.; Pye, R.J.; Kreiss, A.; Cheng, Y.; Brown, G.K.; Darby, J.M.; Malley, R.C.; Siddle, H.V.T.; Skjodt, K.; Kaufman, J.; et al. Regression of devil facial tumor disease following immunotherapy in immunised Tasmanian devils. *Sci. Rep.* **2017**, *7*. [CrossRef] [PubMed]
57. Pye, R.; Patchett, A.; McLennan, E.; Thomson, R.; Carver, S.; Fox, S.; Pemberton, D.; Kreiss, A.; Baz Morelli, A.; Silva, A.; et al. Immunization strategies producing a humoral IgG immune response against Devil Facial Tumor Disease in the majority of Tasmanian devils destined for wild release. *Front. Immunol.* **2018**, *9*, 259. [CrossRef] [PubMed]
58. Lindsey, B.B.; Armitage, E.P.; Kampmann, B.; de Silva, T.I. The efficacy, effectiveness, and immunogenicity of influenza vaccines in Africa: A systematic review. *Lancet Infect. Dis.* **2019**, *19*, e110–e119. [CrossRef]
59. World Health Organization. Q&A on the Malaria Vaccine Implementation Programme (MVIP). Available online: https://www.who.int/malaria/media/malaria-vaccine-implementation-qa/en/ (accessed on 25 November 2019).
60. Long, C.A.; Zavala, F. Malaria vaccines and human immune responses. *Curr. Opin. Microbiol.* **2016**, *32*, 96–102. [CrossRef]

61. Brown, G.K.; Kreiss, A.; Lyons, A.B.; Woods, G.M. Natural killer cell mediated cytotoxic responses in the Tasmanian devil. *PLoS ONE* **2011**, *6*, e24475. [CrossRef]
62. van der Kraan, L.E.; Wong, E.S.; Lo, N.; Ujvari, B.; Belov, K. Identification of natural killer cell receptor genes in the genome of the marsupial Tasmanian devil (*Sarcophilus harrisii*). *Immunogenetics* **2013**, *65*, 25–35. [CrossRef]
63. Saito, F.; Hirayasu, K.; Satoh, T.; Wang, C.W.; Lusingu, J.; Arimori, T.; Shida, K.; Palacpac, N.M.Q.; Itagaki, S.; Iwanaga, S.; et al. Immune evasion of Plasmodium falciparum by RIFIN via inhibitory receptors. *Nature* **2017**, *552*, 101–105. [CrossRef]
64. Caldwell, A.; Coleby, R.; Tovar, C.; Stammnitz, M.R.; Kwon, Y.M.; Owen, R.S.; Tringides, M.; Murchison, E.P.; Skjodt, K.; Thomas, G.J.; et al. The newly-arisen devil facial tumor disease 2 (DFT2) reveals a mechanism for the emergence of a contagious cancer. *eLife* **2018**, *7*. [CrossRef] [PubMed]
65. Kreiss, A.; Tovar, C.; Obendorf, D.L.; Dun, K.; Woods, G.M. A murine xenograft model for a transmissible cancer in Tasmanian devils. *Vet. Pathol.* **2011**, *48*, 475–481. [CrossRef]
66. Mideo, N.; Reece, S.E. Plasticity in parasite phenotypes: Evolutionary and ecological implications for disease. *Future Microbiol.* **2012**, *7*, 17–24. [CrossRef]
67. Maley, C.C.; Aktipis, A.; Graham, T.A.; Sottoriva, A.; Boddy, A.M.; Janiszewska, M.; Silva, A.S.; Gerlinger, M.; Yuan, Y.; Pienta, K.J.; et al. Classifying the evolutionary and ecological features of neoplasms. *Nat. Rev. Cancer* **2017**, *17*, 605–619. [CrossRef] [PubMed]
68. Merlo, L.M.; Pepper, J.W.; Reid, B.J.; Maley, C.C. Cancer as an evolutionary and ecological process. *Nat. Rev. Cancer* **2006**, *6*, 924–935. [CrossRef] [PubMed]
69. Flavahan, W.A.; Gaskell, E.; Bernstein, B.E. Epigenetic plasticity and the hallmarks of cancer. *Science* **2017**, *357*. [CrossRef]
70. Jones, M.E.; Cockburn, A.; Hamede, R.; Hawkins, C.; Hesterman, H.; Lachish, S.; Mann, D.; McCallum, H.; Pemberton, D. Life-history change in disease-ravaged Tasmanian devil populations. *Proc. Natl. Acad. Sci. USA* **2008**, *105*, 10023–10027. [CrossRef]
71. Russell, T.; Madsen, T.; Thomas, F.; Raven, N.; Hamede, R.; Ujvari, B. Oncogenesis as a Selective Force: Adaptive Evolution in the Face of a Transmissible Cancer. *Bioessays* **2018**, *40*. [CrossRef]
72. Ostrander, E.A.; Davis, B.W.; Ostrander, G.K. Transmissible Tumors: Breaking the Cancer Paradigm. *Trends Genet.* **2016**, *32*, 1–15. [CrossRef]
73. Lun, Z.R.; Lai, D.H.; Wen, Y.Z.; Zheng, L.L.; Shen, J.L.; Yang, T.B.; Zhou, W.L.; Qu, L.H.; Hide, G.; Ayala, F.J. Cancer in the parasitic protozoans Trypanosoma brucei and Toxoplasma gondii. *Proc. Natl. Acad. Sci. USA* **2015**, *112*, 8835–8842. [CrossRef]

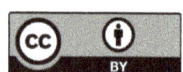

© 2020 by the authors. Licensee MDPI, Basel, Switzerland. This article is an open access article distributed under the terms and conditions of the Creative Commons Attribution (CC BY) license (http://creativecommons.org/licenses/by/4.0/).

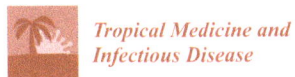

Article

Semi-Quantitative, Duplexed qPCR Assay for the Detection of *Leishmania* spp. Using Bisulphite Conversion Technology

Ineka Gow [1,2,*], Douglas Millar [2], John Ellis [1], John Melki [2] and Damien Stark [3]

1. School of Life Sciences, University of Technology, Sydney, NSW 2007, Australia; john.ellis@uts.edu.au
2. Genetic Signatures Ltd., Sydney, NSW 2042, Australia; doug@geneticsignatures.com (D.M.); john@geneticsignatures.com (J.M.)
3. Microbiology Department, St. Vincent's Hospital, Sydney, NSW 2010, Australia; damien.stark@svha.org.au
* Correspondence: ineka.c.gow@student.uts.edu.au; +61-466263511

Received: 6 October 2019; Accepted: 28 October 2019; Published: 1 November 2019

Abstract: Leishmaniasis is caused by the flagellated protozoan *Leishmania*, and is a neglected tropical disease (NTD), as defined by the World Health Organisation (WHO). Bisulphite conversion technology converts all genomic material to a simplified form during the lysis step of the nucleic acid extraction process, and increases the efficiency of multiplex quantitative polymerase chain reaction (qPCR) reactions. Through utilization of qPCR real-time probes, in conjunction with bisulphite conversion, a new duplex assay targeting the 18S rDNA gene region was designed to detect all *Leishmania* species. The assay was validated against previously extracted DNA, from seven quantitated DNA and cell standards for pan-*Leishmania* analytical sensitivity data, and 67 cutaneous clinical samples for cutaneous clinical sensitivity data. Specificity was evaluated by testing 76 negative clinical samples and 43 bacterial, viral, protozoan and fungal species. The assay was also trialed in a side-by-side experiment against a conventional PCR (cPCR), based on the Internal transcribed spacer region 1 (ITS1 region). Ninety-seven percent of specimens from patients that previously tested positive for *Leishmania* were positive for *Leishmania spp.* with the bisulphite conversion assay, and a limit of detection (LOD) of 10 copies per PCR was achieved, while the LOD of the ITS1 methodology was 10 cells/1000 genomic copies per PCR. This method of rapid, accurate and simple detection of *Leishmania* can lead to improved diagnosis, treatment and public health outcomes.

Keywords: leishmaniasis; qPCR; bisulphite

1. Introduction

Leishmaniasis is an infection caused by some species of *Leishmania* parasites that affect the skin, organs and mucosal regions of the body, leading to serious morbidity and possibly death. It is classed as a Neglected Tropical Disease (NTD), affecting 12 million people worldwide, with a further 350 million people at risk of contracting the disease [1]. With the advent of increased human international travel, due to work, tourism or war, leishmaniasis is now an emerging infectious disease, with an increased impact on global mortality and morbidity [2]. It is becoming increasingly clear that there is a need for accurate and rapid detection of *Leishmania* in the form of a standardized and validated assay, to aid diagnosis, treatment and surveillance programs.

Many validated molecular *Leishmania* detection assays use conventional PCR (cPCR) for the detection of *Leishmania* infection [3–5]. Conventional PCR is a diagnostic method where DNA is amplified using a thermal cycler, amplicons are separated due to molecular weight by electrophoresis, and detected by stain (usually ethidium bromide or gel red) and UV light (via a transilluminator) [6]. This approach requires significantly more hands-on time, has a greater risk of contamination and makes multiplexing analysis more difficult if products are similar in size, compared to real-time PCR. Probe-based qPCR can overcome these issues. Additionally, specificity can be increased, and it allows for continuous monitoring of the PCR. The 18S rRNA gene (18S rDNA) is a highly conserved gene across all *Leishmania* species, despite having diverged from other similarly related species during the period Paleogene or Paleocene [7]. The gene exists in between 50–200 copies per *Leishmania* genome, making it an excellent choice for a pan-*Leishmania* detection assay [6]. To assess whether this target can be used in a novel diagnostic assay, based on bisulphite conversion and real-time PCR technologies, a series of experiments were performed to assess the limit of detection and sensitivity of the assay, and the new assay was compared to a cPCR, based on the ITS1 region, developed by Schönian et al. [8].

The development of this novel bisulphite-converted, qPCR assay methodology, based on genus-specific primer and probe designs for the 18S rDNA, and its validation, is described in this paper. Furthermore, the bisulphite conversion and purification of protozoan DNA are discussed. The assay's limit of detection was 10 cellular or genomic copies/PCR, with clinical sensitivity and specificity demonstrated to be 97.0% and 100%, respectively. The assay takes under 2.5 hours to complete, making the assay a potential diagnostic tool for both diagnostic and research laboratories worldwide.

2. Materials and Methods

2.1. Specimens Tested

DNA was purified from cell-cultured promastigotes of the following species: *L. donovani* (MHOM/IN/80/DD8 supplied at 2.3×10^7 cells/mL), *L. braziliensis* (MHOM/BR/75/M2903 supplied at 1.63×10^8 cells/mL), *L. tropica* (MHOM/SU/74/K27 supplied at 1.03×10^7 cells/mL), *L. amazonensis* (MHOM/BR/73/M2269 supplied at 9.9×10^6 cells/mL), *L. mexicana* (MHOM/BZ/82/BEL21 supplied at 1.51×10^8 cells/mL) and *L. major* (MHOM/SU/73/5-ASKH supplied at 7.1×10^6 cells/mL), obtained from the American type culture collection (ATCC, Manassas, USA). *Leishmania infantum* genomic DNA (supplied at 1.2×10^7 copies/mL) was obtained from Vircell (Vircell, Granada, Spain). The assay was initially evaluated by performing a 10-fold serial dilution series of the DNA from these strains to assess the limit of detection. In addition, DNA from 67 previously extracted cutaneous clinical samples (derived from 66 unique patients), that were previously identified by St. Vincent's Hospital, Sydney as positive for *Leishmania* by the cPCR method, during the period 2007–2016, were included in the study [8–10]. All DNA was initially extracted using the EZ1 tissue kit on the EZ1 biorobot (Qiagen, Hilden, Germany), in accordance with manufacturers' recommendations regarding direct sample or following culture. Specificity was assessed by extracting DNA using standard methods from 76 negative tissue samples, previously characterised at St. Vincent's Hospital, Sydney, and 43 potential cross-reacting organisms, and testing them in the assay (Table 1). The clinical specimens were tested in accordance with St Vincent's Hospital ethics approval, HREC number LNR/16/SVH/231.

Table 1. List of organisms used in this study for cross-reactivity testing for the novel bisulphite conversion assay.

Specimen Number	Organism
1	*Acinetobacter baumanni*
2	*Bacillus cereus*
3	*Bacillus subtilis*
4	*Clostridium perfringens*
5	*Clostridium sordelli*
6	*Escherichia coli*

Table 1. *Cont.*

Specimen Number	Organism
7	*Haemophilus influenzae*
8	*Klebsiella oxytoca*
9	*Klebsiella pneumoniae*
10	*Moraxella cattaharalis*
11	*Proteus mirabilis*
12	*Proteus vulgaris*
13	*Pseudomonas aeruginosa*
14	*Staphylococcus aureus*
15	*Staphylococcus hominis*
16	*Streptococcus pyogenes*
17	*Streptococcus sp. (mutans)*
18	*Yersinia sp.*
19	*Mycobacteria abscessus*
20	*Mycobacteria marinum*
21	*Mycobacteria sp.*
22	Herpes Simplex Virus Type I
23	Herpes Simplex Virus Type II
24	Varicella Zoster Virus
25	*Trichophyton tonsurans*
26	*Trichophyton mentagrophytes*
27	*Microsporum canis*
28	*Aspergillus fumigatus*
29	*Acromium pulluans*
30	*Acromium strictum*
31	*Aspergillus sp.*
32	*Bipolaris sp.*
33	*Fusarium sp.*
34	*Penicillium sp.*
35	*Scedosporium prolificans*
36	*Trichophyton rubrum*
37	Bovine
38	Human
39	*Trypanosoma cruzi*
40	*Crithidia lucilae*
41	*Trichomonas vaginalis*
42	*Giardia intestinalis*
43	*Entamoeba histolytica*

2.2. DNA Conversion and Quality Control

Genomic DNA was bisulphite converted by adding 2,880,000 or 28,800 copies of DNA/cellular standards, depending on available starting concentration, to a total volume of 150 µL with molecular grade H$_2$O, then adding 250 µL 3M sodium bisulphite. Alternatively, 5 µL of DNA, previously extracted from cutaneous clinical sample DNA, were added to 145 µL of molecular grade H$_2$O, then 250 µL 3M sodium bisulphite was added. One negative process control of 150 µL molecular grade H$_2$O was included in each run, to check for contamination. A total of 5×10^5 copies/µL Lambda DNA (strain cI857 ind 1 Sam 7) (New England Biolabs, Ipswich, USA), an *Escherichia coli* bacteriophage, was added to each of these reactions, then the samples were mixed by vortexing, and incubated at 95 °C for 15 minutes. Subsequently 200 µL of this lysate was purified on the GS-mini (Genetic Signatures Ltd., Sydney, Australia) with the Sample Processing Pathogens A kit (Genetic Signatures Ltd., Sydney, Australia), according to the manufacturers' recommendations. The eluted DNA was then diluted in molecular grade H$_2$O in 10-fold dilution series, to 0.1 copy per PCR. The limit of detection (LOD) for this study was defined as the lowest concentration of DNA at which the assay detected 10 out of 10 replicates, in accordance with CLSI standards, which define the LOD as the lowest dilution where 95% of replicates are positive [11]. Cell and DNA concentrations were provided by the suppliers and copy number was calculated (https://www.thermofisher.com/au/en/home/brands/thermo-scientific/molecular-biology/molecular-biology-learning-center/molecular-biology-resource-library/thermo-scientific-web-tools/dna-copy-number-calculator.html). The GS-mini employs a closed cartridge-based system, whereby nucleic acid is bound to magnetic beads, with subsequent washing and, finally, elution steps, using heating and shaking to increase nucleic acid yield. Separate PCR areas were used for mastermix preparation, DNA seeding and PCR reactions, to prevent the possibility of PCR contamination. The addition of lambda bacteriophage DNA to the PCR reaction was used to monitor the efficiency of the bisulphite conversion, purification, and in assessing for possible false negatives due to PCR inhibition. A negative process control (molecular grade H$_2$O) controlled for possible PCR contamination.

An external positive control was developed by creating a geneblock—a synthetic double stranded 1000bp-long fragment of the 18S rDNA of *L. donovani*, (GenBank accession CP022642 positions 1047751 to 1048750), consisting of adenine, thymine, cytosine or guanine residues only. This was bisulphite converted and diluted to five copies/µL in molecular grade H$_2$O, using the previously described protocol.

2.3. PCR Primer and Probe Design

For the 18S rDNA assay forward, reverse primers and a probe were designed, based on multiple sequence alignments of the 18S rDNA in bisulphite converted form (that is, with all cytosines converted to thymines), of the species *Leishmania aethiopica*, *Leishmania amazonensis*, *Leishmania braziliensis*, *Leishmania colombiensis*, *Leishmania donovani*, *Leishmania guyanensis*, *Leishmania infantum*, *Leishmania lainsoni*, *Leishmania major*, *Leishmania mexicana*, *Leishmania naiffi*, *Leishmania panamensis*, *Leishmania shawi* and *Leishmania tropica*. This resulted in the identification of primers PL-18S-F2 (TTATTGTTTTGGTTTTTG) and PL-18S-R2 (AAACCAAAATTACAATAAAA) and probe PL-18S-P2 (GGAGATTATGGAGTTGTGTGATA), which amplify and detect DNA fragments of 82bp in length. The exogenous control was targeted by primers Lambda New F1 (AATATTGGTAGATTATGTTTGTG), Lambda New R1 (CTATCATCAAATCATACAATACC) and probe Lambda New P1 (TGATGTGATAGGAAGAATTTGTTGTTGTTGTTGTTG), which amplify a 100bp fragment of the Lambda bacteriophage DNA. The 18S rDNA and Lambda probes are intercalating, self-quenching probes, labeled with individual fluorophores (FAM and HEX, respectively) enabling the PCR to be performed as a duplex reaction.

2.4. PCR Preparation, Conditions, and Interpretation

The PCR mixture was prepared by using 10µL of 2x SensiFast (Bioline), 90ng of each primer PL-18S-F2/PL-18S-R2 and 8 pmol probe PL-18S-P2, 4ng primer Lambda New F1, 40ng primer Lambda New R1 and 3pmol probe Lambda New P1, 3.5µL of template, and molecular grade H_2O, to a final volume of 20µl. All DNA templates were tested in 10 PCR replicates. A negative template control reaction was included in each PCR run. PCRs were run on the MIC PCR thermal cycler (Bio Molecular Systems, Upper Coomera, Australia) using the following parameters: 95 °C for 3 min, and 50 cycles of 95 °C for 2 s and 50 °C for 10 s, 55 °C for 10 s (data acquisition step) and 60 °C for 10 s.

The new assay was tested against the Schönian method by processing the equivalent concentration of *Leishmania* cells or genomic DNA, diluting these in molecular grade H_2O, and heating at 70 °C for 15 minutes. Next, these lysates were processed on the GS-mini, using the MagPurix Viral/Pathogen Nucleic Acids Extraction Kit (Zinexts Life Science, Taipei, Taiwan) on the GS-mini, following the manufacturers' instructions. The eluates were diluted in the same fashion as the bisulphite-treated eluates and amplified in cPCR triplicates, according to the methodology developed by Schönian et al., with primers LITSR: CTGGATCATTTTCCGATG and L5.8S: TGATACCACTTATCGCACTT (targeting the ssu rRNA and 5.8S rRNA, respectively) [8].

3. Results

3.1. Specificity of the Real-Time PCR Assay Using Quantitated Cultured Cell or Purified DNA Standards

DNA converted from the panel of seven *Leishmania* quantitated standards (*L. donovani, L. braziliensis, L. tropica, L. amazonensis, L. major, L. mexicana* and *L. infantum*) were detected by the 18S rDNA assay (Table 2). As displayed in Table 2, there was a concordance between these results and the Schönian method, as all *Leishmania* species tested were detected [8].

Table 2. Detection limit of the conventional and novel PCR assays.

Species	Supplier	Schönian Method	Novel Method
L. donovani	ATCC	100 cells/PCR	10 cells/PCR
L. braziliensis	ATCC	100 cells/PCR	10 cells/PCR
L. tropica	ATCC	100 cells/PCR	10 cells/PCR
L. amazonensis	ATCC	100 cells/PCR	10 cells/PCR
L. mexicana	ATCC	100 cells/PCR	100 cells/PCR
L. major	ATCC	10 cells/PCR	10 cells/PCR
L. infantum	Vircell	1000 copies/PCR	10 copies/PCR

3.2. Specificity of the Real-Time PCR Assay Using Negative Control Samples

DNA, extracted from 76 negative clinical samples, did not produce any PCR products using the new assay, giving a specificity of 100% [8].

3.3. Specificity of the Real-Time PCR Assay Using Cross-Reactivity Specimens

To further investigate the specificity of the assay, a panel of DNA from 43 other phylogenetically related organisms, or those with a differential diagnosis related to leishmaniasis, was tested (Table 1). No PCR products were detected from any of these specimens, giving a specificity of 100%.

3.4. Limit of Detection of the Real-Time PCR Assay Using Quantitated Standards

The analytical sensitivity of the assay was evaluated using quantitated DNA and cell culture standards. Ten-fold serial dilutions were tested in the assay, and the LOD for *Leishmania* was shown to be 10 cellular/genomic copies per PCR reaction, although this LOD differed between species, as outlined in Table 2. For *L. braziliensis*, for example, the LOD was 10 cellular copies, and an average of 38.7 cycle threshold (C_T) value was determined after testing the sample in 10 PCR replicates. When *L. braziliensis* was tested by the Schönian method, the LOD was 100 cellular copies/PCR when tested in triplicate (Figure 1). ATCC quantitation was given in cells/μL and Vircell quantitation was given in copies/μL, so this nomenclature has been upheld.

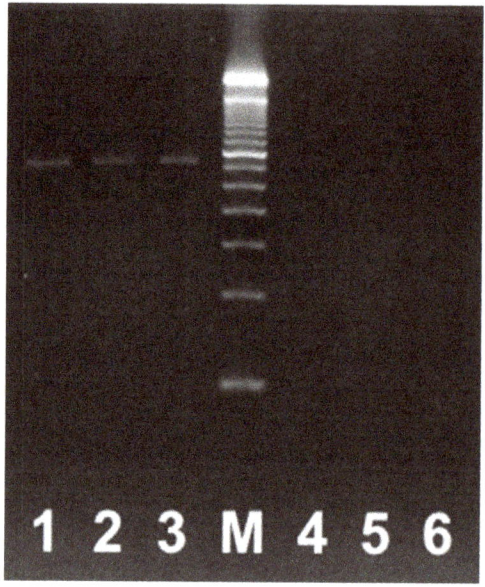

Figure 1. Sensitivity of the ITS1 cPCR assay for *L. braziliensis*, gel electrophoresis of conventional PCR result, using the Schönian method. Lanes 1, 2 and 3 are 100 copies/PCR; lane M is the 100bp ladder size standard, lanes 4, 5 and 6 are 10 copies/PCR.

3.5. Sensitivity of the Real-Time PCR Assay Using Clinical Sample DNA

Previously extracted DNA from 67 clinical tissue samples was available from patients with confirmed diagnosis of cutaneous leishmaniasis. Although clinical data were not available for all specimens, of those samples with data available, 32 (72.7%) were male, and the age range was between one and 73 years. Forty-two patients had data available on previous travel; 21 (50.0%) of these patients had been to the middle east, 11 (26.2%) had been to South America, three (7.1%) had been to southern Europe, one (2.4%) to South Asia and five patients (11.9%) had been to multiple geographic regions. Reason for travel data were available for 39 patients; 26 (66.7%) were travellers, nine were immigrants (28.2%) and two (5.1%) were members of the army. Resulting cPCR (Schönian method) and restriction fragment length polymorphism analysis were used for detection and species differentiation, respectively [8]. Of the 67 clinical samples, the novel assay was detected in 65, thus 97.0 % concordance was achieved between the previous method and the 18S assay.

3.6. Precision of the Real-Time PCR Assay Using Quantitated Standards

Standard curves were produced for *L. braziliensis* and *L. tropica*, testing 10-fold serial dilutions in PCR triplicates, giving an R^2 value of 0.9945 for *L. braziliensis* (Figure 2a,b). This is a measure of the linearity of the generated curves and reflects efficiency and reproducibility. Error bars depict 95% confidence intervals, based upon two experimental replicates, comprising three PCR technical replicates each. To measure the intra-experiment precision and agreement between experiments, five experiments were each performed over five consecutive days, with three replicates at two cellular concentrations for each species (Table 3). The results considered over 236 replicates, with four negative replicates for *L. tropica* excluded. Low coefficients of variation (CVs), related to intra-experiment variability, were observed, all <10%. These findings provide additional support that this novel, real-time PCR provides efficient and precise quantification of DNA within and between experiments.

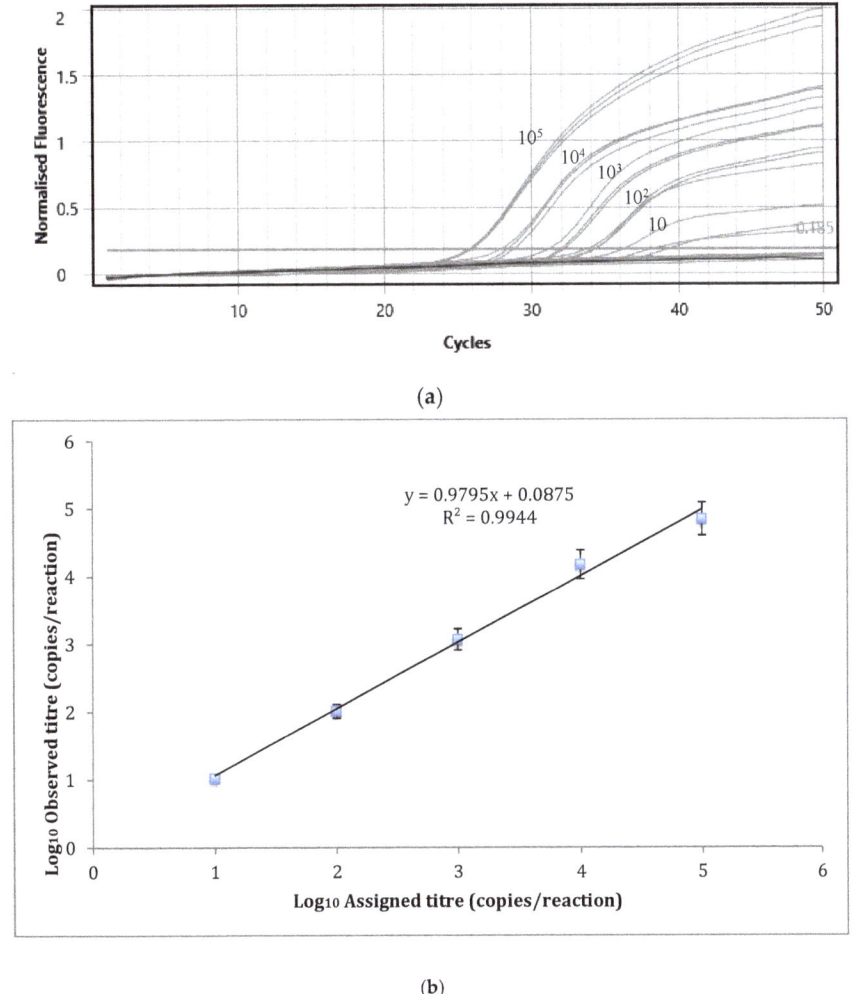

(a)

(b)

Figure 2. Sensitivity of the novel qPCR assay for *L. braziliensis*. (**a**) FAM channel amplification curves, using 10-fold serial dilutions from 10^5 to 0.1 copies per PCR, tested in PCR triplicate. (**b**) Graphic depiction of the linear range of detection (10 to 10^5 copies per reaction). Error bars represent 95% CI.

Table 3. Summary of the Observed Precision Estimates for the novel assay.

Leishmania Species and Copy Number	Mean (Ct)	SD (Ct)	CV (%)
L. donovani 1000 c/PCR	30.26	0.88	2.92
L. donovani 100 c/PCR	33.28	0.99	2.98
L. braziliensis 100 c/PCR	30.78	0.87	2.84
L. braziliensis 10 c/PCR	33.71	0.67	1.99
L. tropica 100 c/PCR	34.07	0.95	2.80
L. tropica 10 c/PCR[1]	37.83	2.31	6.11
L. amazonensis 100 c/PCR	31.29	1.09	3.50
L. amazonensis 10 c/PCR	34.24	2.19	6.39
L. mexicana 1000 c/PCR	33.08	1.19	3.61
L. mexicana 100 c/PCR	36.22	1.52	4.19
L. major 100 c/PCR	31.96	0.84	2.62
L. major 10 c/PCR	35.09	0.74	2.10
L. infantum 1000 c/PCR	29.44	1.22	4.13
L. infantum 100 c/PCR	32.23	1.47	4.57

[1] For *L. tropica*, only 2/3 replicates were achieved on four of the five consecutive days tested. In order to assess mean, SD and CV, the negative data points were excluded from the data set.

3.7. Internal Control Reaction

No samples showed inhibition of the exogenous control.

4. Discussion

The development of a multiplexed, real-time PCR, targeting the 18S rDNA to detect all *Leishmania* species and the associated automated bisulphite conversion system, is described. The assay was validated on DNA and cell standards and the limit of detection, using seven individual strains of *Leishmania*. The LOD was compared with the method of Schönian et al. [8] and, as can be seen from Table 2, the LOD of all seven species improved upon using the real-time PCR method [8]. No cross-reactivity was observed using a panel of 43 possible cross-reacting organisms (Table 1) and 76 negative tissue samples, making the assay exclusive to *Leishmania* DNA detection. For clinical performance, the DNA of 67 previously described positive tissue samples were tested, alongside a conventional PCR method, as described by Schönian et al., and 65 samples tested positive in the 18S rDNA real-time PCR assay [8]. The Schönian method is based on the ITS1 region, a gene also located on the ribosomal DNA array, and thus present in the same number of copies as the 18S rRNA gene [12]. The novel assay includes an exogenous control, which controls for extraction and PCR performance, and an external positive control, controlling for PCR performance. The inclusion of quality controls, both internal and external, was highlighted as important in *Leishmania* detection assays [13]. The turn-around time is less than 2.5 hours from sample to result, and the system has a small laboratory footprint (the area required in the laboratory for instrumentation) of 75cm by 75cm.

The assay is based on the gene coding for the small subunit rRNA, a highly conserved region of the ribosomal DNA, located on chromosome 27. This gene was used for the detection of *Leishmania* in other assays, due to its excellent sensitivity, attributed to the fact that it is a multicopy gene, which is transcribed into abundant rRNA found in the cytoplasm, where it is predicted to be present at 10^4 copies [7,14–16].

The test utilises bisulphite conversion technology, whereby the genome is simplified to three nucleobases: A, T and G (Figure S1). This simplification of the genome enables easier design of primers and probes across subtypes and species variants, as single oligonucleotide sets can be designed to cover a diverse population and reduce the need for multiplexing, in order to capture all species. Furthermore, the increase in homology allows for different primer and probe sets of differing targets to be designed with similar melting temperatures (Tm), reducing potential issues with specificity (Table S1). This was previously demonstrated in two clinical trials, where nearly 100% sensitivity and specificity were achieved by the increased homology and similar Tm of the primers and probes designed for the assays [17,18]. Bisulphite conversion technology is already in use in various diagnostic laboratories in the detection of clinical sample types, including gastro-intestinal infections [18,19]. The bisulphite conversion is included in the initial lysis step and therefore requires no extra steps by the end user. This is the first *Leishmania* detection assay exploiting bisulphite technology. The bisulphite conversion technology can also be used in an assay designed to differentiate *Leishmania* species. As there are over 20 *Leishmania* species pathogenic to humans, these will need to be multiplexed with up to four other targets into at least five panels [20]. A similar Tm greatly reduces the risk of non-specific amplification, as a lower melting temperature can be used across the PCR cycling protocol, but will accommodate all targets. In this way, a future assay may be designed to incorporate the novel pan-*Leishmania* assay to screen a given sample, then a reflex assay may be used to identify the causative *Leishmania* species. In intercalating self-quenching probes, such as those used in this assay, the fluorescent dye and quencher are at separate ends, that are in a hairpin conformation when not bound to target [21]. This gives less non-specific fluorescence, as the probe is in close proximity to the quencher, and, thus, is more effectively quenched.(See Supplementary Materials)

Leishmania DNA-based detection in the laboratory is dominated by cPCR, nested PCR or qPCR. Conventional PCR has sensitivities ranging from 56% to 100%, depending on clinical specimen and gene target [8,22]. In nested PCR, an inner and outer set of primers are designed and tested in two rounds to increase sensitivity and specificity [23]. In an Iranian study of cutaneous leishmaniasis patients, it gave a sensitivity of 100% [24]. Both these methods, however, are time-consuming and laborious, requiring gel electrophoresis and a transilluminator for imaging post-PCR. This may also leave the laboratory open to contamination risk during these post-PCR methods. Quantitative PCR is a closed-tube system, where one step is required between DNA addition and result, and results may be read in real-time [25]. It achieves sensitivities and specificities of up to 100% [26,27]. The novel qPCR achieved a lower LOD than cPCR, an outcome seen in other *Leishmania* assays utilising various targets [14,28,29]. Our future studies will determine the clinical sensitivity of samples previously tested positive for visceral leishmaniasis, to complement the clinical data obtained here.

Currently, there are very few commercial assays available on the market for the detection of all *Leishmania* species, particularly those based on the detection of *Leishmania* DNA, however, no formal evaluations are described in the scientific literature. Primer Design provide a primer and probe set with mastermix and controls, which claims to detect all *Leishmania* species, based on the cytochrome b gene. This is a qPCR test, providing lyophilized components, with a sensitivity of 100 copies (http://www.genesig.com/assets/files/leishmania_spp_std.pdf). Another assay detects *L. major* only (MyBioSource), through a qPCR assay containing the primers, probes, mastermix and controls. It claims a sensitivity of 100 copies of target template (https://www.mybiosource.com/images/tds/protocol_manuals/000000-799999/MBS486088_Easy.pdf). BioKits have a cPCR kit detection *Leishmania* spp., containing ready-to-use PCR mix and positive control, with a sensitivity of 20 copies/mL (http://www.biokits.com/productinfo/3587/Leishmania-sp.-PCR-Detection-Kit.html). The US army has an FDA-approved *Leishmania* qPCR detection kit called SMART Leish, developed in conjunction with Cepheid and the Walter Reed Army Institute of Research for the diagnosis of species associated with cutaneous leishmaniasis, with an LOD of four genome copies (http://www.accessdata.fda.gov/cdrh_docs/pdf8/K081868.pdf). Its use is restricted to the Department of Defense laboratories, and thus not available commercially.

The novel pan-*Leishmania* assay provides a simple, economical solution for a high-tech molecular detection system, while retaining excellent sensitivity and specificity, that can be easily used in reference and satellite laboratories alike. Moreover, the automated nature of this system and its low cost means its application is feasible in many countries where leishmaniasis is endemic, which may lack the finances and expertise to implement high-tech laboratory diagnostics, such as qPCR. Such an efficient workflow and quality performance assures that reliable patient results can be diagnosed quickly, treatment regimes can be administered, and prognosis can be assessed.

Supplementary Materials: The following are available online at http://www.mdpi.com/2414-6366/4/4/135/s1, Figure S1: Conventional and bisulphite converted alignments for the 18S rDNA gene, Table S1: Conventional and bisulphite converted primer and probe designs for the novel assay.

Author Contributions: Conceptualization, I.G., D.S., D.M. and J.E.; methodology, I.G.; validation, I.G.; formal analysis, I.G.; investigation, I.G.; resources, J.M.; data curation, I.G.; writing—original draft preparation, I.G.; writing—review and editing, D.S., D.M. and J.E; visualization, I.G.; supervision, D.S.; project administration, I.G.; funding acquisition, J.M.

Funding: This research received no external funding

Acknowledgments: We are grateful to Rogan Lee for the supply of *Leishmania*.

Conflicts of Interest: DM, IG and JM are employees of Genetic Signatures Ltd.

References

1. World Health Organisation. *Control of the Leishmaniases*; WHO Technical Report Series 949; World Health Organisation: Geneva, Switzerland, 2010.
2. Hotez, P.J. Human Parasitology and Parasitic Diseases: Heading Towards. *Adv. Parasitol.* **2018**, *100*, 29–38. [PubMed]
3. Gualda, K.P.; Marcussi, L.M.; Neitzke-Abreu, H.C.; Aristides, S.M.A.; Lonardoni, M.V.C.; Cardoso, R.F.; Silveira, T.G.V. New Primers for Detection of *Leishmania infantum* using Polymerase Chain Reaction. *Rev. Inst. Med. Trop. Sao Paulo* **2015**, *57*, 377–383. [CrossRef] [PubMed]
4. Ranasinghe, S.; Wickremasinghe, R.; Hulangamuwa, S.; Sirimanna, G.; Opathella, N.; Maingon, R.D.; Chandrasekharan, V. Polymerase chain reaction detection of Leishmania DNA in skin biopsy samples in Sri Lanka where the causative agent of cutaneous leishmaniasis is Leishmania donovani. *Memórias Inst. Oswaldo. Cruz* **2015**, *110*, 1017–1023. [CrossRef] [PubMed]
5. De Cassia-Pires, R.; de Melo, M.F.; Barbosa, R.D.; Roque, A.L. Multiplex PCR as a tool for the diagnosis of Leishmania skDNA and the gapdh housekeeping gene of mammal hosts. *PLoS ONE* **2017**, *12*, e0173922. [CrossRef]
6. Srivastava, P.; Mehrotra, S.; Tiwary, P.; Chakravarty, J.; Sundar, S. Diagnosis of Indian Visceral Leishmaniasis by Nucleic Acid Detection Using PCR. *PLoS ONE* **2011**, *6*, e19304. [CrossRef]
7. Tuon, F.F.; Neto, V.A.; Amato, V.S. Leishmania: origin, evolution and future since the Precambrian. *FEMS Immunol. Med. Microbiol.* **2008**, *54*, 158–166. [CrossRef]
8. Schönian, G.; Nasereddin, A.; Dinse, N.; Schweynoch, C.; Schallig, H.D.F.H.; Presber, W.; Jaffe, C.L. PCR diagnosis and characterization of Leishmania in local and imported clinical samples. *Diagn. Microbiol. Infect. Dis.* **2003**, *47*, 349–358. [CrossRef]
9. Roberts, T.; Barratt, J.; Sandaradura, I.; Lee, R.; Harkness, J.; Marriott, D.; Ellis, J.; Stark, D. Molecular Epidemiology of Imported Cases of Leishmaniasis in Australia from 2008 to 2014. *PLoS ONE* **2015**, *10*, e0119212. [CrossRef]
10. Lee, R.; Marriott, D.; Stark, D.; Van Hal, S.; Harkness, J. Leishmaniasis, an Emerging Imported Infection: Report of 20 Cases from Australia: Table. *J. Travel Med.* **2008**, *15*, 351–354.
11. Larrisey, M.P. *EP17-A2 Evaluation of Detection Capability for Clinical Laboratory Measurement Procedures. Approved Guideline—Second Edition*; Clinical and Laboratory Standards Institute: Wayne, PA, USA, 2012; pp. 2–18.
12. Töz, S.; Özensoy; Çulha, G.; Zeyrek, F.Y.; Ertabaklar, H.; Alkan, M.Z.; Vardarlı, A.T.; Gunduz, C.; Özbel, Y. A Real-Time ITS1-PCR Based Method in the Diagnosis and Species Identification of Leishmania Parasite from Human and Dog Clinical Samples in Turkey. *PLoS Neglected Trop. Dis.* **2013**, *7*, e2205.
13. Gonçalves-de-Albuquerque, S.D.C.; Pessoa-e-Silva, R.; Trajano-Silva, L.A.M.; de Morais, R.C.S.; Brandao-Filho, S.P.; de Paiva-Cavalcanti, M. Inclusion of quality controls on leishmaniases molecular tests to increase diagnostic accuracy in research and reference laboratories. *Mol. Biotechnol.* **2015**, *57*, 318–324. [CrossRef] [PubMed]

14. León, C.M.; Muñoz, M.; Hernández, C.; Ayala, M.S.; Flórez, C.; Teherán, A.; Cubides, J.R.; Ramírez, J.D. Analytical Performance of Four Polymerase Chain Reaction (PCR) and Real Time PCR (qPCR) Assays for the Detection of Six Leishmania Species DNA in Colombia. *Front. Microbiol.* **2017**, *8*, 8. [CrossRef] [PubMed]
15. Vaish, M.; Mehrotra, S.; Chakravarty, J.; Sundar, S. Noninvasive Molecular Diagnosis of Human Visceral Leishmaniasis. *J. Clin. Microbiol.* **2011**, *49*, 2003–2005. [CrossRef] [PubMed]
16. Van Eys, G.J.J.M.; Schoone, G.J.; Kroon, N.C.; Ebeling, S.B. Sequence analysis of small subunit ribosomal RNA genes and its use for detection and identification of Leishmania parasites. *Mol. Biochem. Parasitol.* **1992**, *51*, 133–142.
17. Siah, S.P.; Merif, J.; Kaur, K.; Nair, J.; Huntington, P.G.; Karagiannis, T.; Stark, D.; Rawlinson, W.; Olma, T.; Thomas, L.; et al. Improved detection of gastrointestinal pathogens using generalised sample processing and amplification panels. *Pathology* **2014**, *46*, 53–59. [CrossRef]
18. Baleriola, C.; Millar, D.; Melki, J.; Coulston, N.; Altman, P.; Rismanto, N.; Rawlinson, W. Comparison of a novel HPV test with the Hybrid Capture II (hcII) and a reference PCR method shows high specificity and positive predictive value for 13 high-risk human papillomavirus infections. *J. Clin. Virol.* **2008**, *42*, 22–26. [CrossRef]
19. Stark, D.; Roberts, T.; Ellis, J.; Marriott, D.; Harkness, J. Evaluation of the EasyScreen™ Enteric Parasite Detection Kit for the detection of Blastocystis spp., Cryptosporidium spp., Dientamoeba fragilis, Entamoeba complex, and Giardia intestinalis from clinical stool samples. *Diagn. Microbiol. Infect. Dis.* **2014**, *78*, 149–152. [CrossRef]
20. Akhoundi, M.; Downing, T.; Votýpka, J.; Kuhls, K.; Lukeš, J.; Cannet, A.; Ravel, C.; Marty, P.; Delaunay, P.; Kasbari, M.; et al. Leishmania infections: Molecular targets and diagnosis. *Mol. Asp. Med.* **2017**, *57*, 1–29. [CrossRef]
21. Kjelland, V.; Stuen, S.; Skarpaas, T.; Slettan, A. Prevalence and genotypes of Borrelia burgdorferi sensu lato infection in Ixodes ricinus ticks in southern Norway. *Scand. J. Infect. Dis.* **2010**, *42*, 579–585. [CrossRef]
22. Saab, M.; El Hage, H.; Charafeddine, K.; Habib, R.H.; Khalifeh, I. Diagnosis of Cutaneous Leishmaniasis: Why Punch When You Can Scrape? *Am. J. Trop. Med. Hyg.* **2015**, *92*, 518–522. [CrossRef]
23. Haddad, M.H.F.; Ghasemi, E.; Maraghi, S.; Tavala, M. Identification of Leishmania Species Isolated from Human Cutaneous Leishmaniasis in Mehran, Western Iran Using Nested PCR. *Iran. J. Parasitol.* **2016**, *11*, 65–72.
24. Namazi, M.J.; Dehkordi, A.B.; Haghighi, F.; Mohammadzadeh, M.; Zarean, M.; Hasanabad, M.H. Molecular detection of Leishmania species in northeast of Iran. *Comp. Haematol. Int.* **2018**, *27*, 729–733. [CrossRef]
25. De Almeida, M.E.; Koru, O.; Steurer, F.; Herwaldt, B.L.; da Silva, A.J. Detection and Differentiation of Leishmania sin Clinical Specimens by Use of a SYBR Green-Based Real-Time PCR Assay. *J Clin. Microbiol.* **2017**, *55*, 281–290. [CrossRef] [PubMed]
26. Mohammadiha, A.; Mohebali, M.; Haghighi, A.; Mahdian, R.; Abadi, A.; Zarei, Z.; Yeganeh, F.; Kazemi, B.; Taghipour, N.; Akhoundi, B. Comparison of real-time PCR and conventional PCR with two DNA targets for detection of Leishmania (Leishmania) infantum infection in human and dog blood samples. *Exp. Parasitol.* **2013**, *133*, 89–94. [CrossRef] [PubMed]
27. Sudarshan, M.; Singh, T.; Chakravarty, J.; Sundar, S. A Correlative Study of Splenic Parasite Score and Peripheral Blood Parasite Load Estimation by Quantitative PCR in Visceral Leishmaniasis. *J. Clin. Microbiol.* **2015**, *53*, 3905–3907. [CrossRef] [PubMed]
28. Sterkers, Y.; Varlet-Marie, E.; Cassaing, S.; Brenier-Pinchart, M.-P.; Brun, S.; Dalle, F.; Delhaes, L.; Filisetti, D.; Pelloux, H.; Yera, H.; et al. Multicentric Comparative Analytical Performance Study for Molecular Detection of Low Amounts of Toxoplasma gondii from Simulated Specimens. *J. Clin. Microbiol.* **2010**, *48*, 3216–3222. [CrossRef]
29. Eroglu, F.; Koltas, I.S.; Uzun, S. Comparison of Clinical Samples and Methods in Chronic Cutaneous Leishmaniasis. *Am. J. Trop. Med. Hyg.* **2014**, *91*, 895–900. [CrossRef]

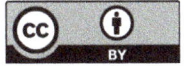 © 2019 by the authors. Licensee MDPI, Basel, Switzerland. This article is an open access article distributed under the terms and conditions of the Creative Commons Attribution (CC BY) license (http://creativecommons.org/licenses/by/4.0/).

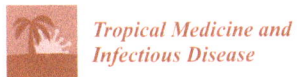

Case Report

Gnathostomiasis Acquired by Visitors to the Okavango Delta, Botswana

John Frean [1,2]

[1] Centre for Emerging Zoonotic and Parasitic Diseases, National Institute for Communicable Diseases, Division of the National Health Laboratory Service, Johannesburg 2192, South Africa; johnf@nicd.ac.za
[2] Wits Research Institute for Malaria, University of the Witwatersrand, Johannesburg 2193, South Africa

Received: 29 January 2020; Accepted: 4 March 2020; Published: 6 March 2020

Abstract: Gnathostomiasis is a zoonotic nematode parasite disease, most commonly acquired by eating raw or undercooked fish. Although the disease is well known in parts of Asia and Central and South America, relatively few cases have been reported from Africa. Raw fish consumed in the Okavango River delta area of Botswana, and in nearby western Zambia, has previously produced laboratory-proven gnathostomiasis in tourists. The purpose of this communication is to record additional cases of the infection acquired in the Okavango delta, and to alert visitors to the inadvisability of eating raw freshwater fish in the southern African region.

Keywords: *Gnathostoma* species; gnathostomiasis; larva migrans; Okavango; southern Africa; tourists

1. Introduction

With the global growth in tourism, increasing numbers of travellers visit what were once remote and unusual destinations, many of which are located in tropical, low-income countries. Immersion in local culture can expose travellers to unusual, often unpleasant, and sometimes dangerous pathogens. This is particularly so when they are food- or water-associated, as visitors cannot easily avoid these vehicles of transmission, or may even pursue them in the interests of adventurous eating. Further increasing the risk of infection, local foods may traditionally be consumed raw or incompletely cooked [1]. Importation or local cultivation of exotic food species may greatly extend the geographic range of associated pathogens [2].

Gnathostoma species are spirurid nematode parasites with a complex transmission cycle involving terrestrial and aquatic hosts (Figure 1), and humans are infected by consuming the intermediate hosts in the form of raw food, usually fish. While gnathostomiasis is well known in parts of Asia and Latin America [3], it is a relatively newly-described culinary risk in Africa.

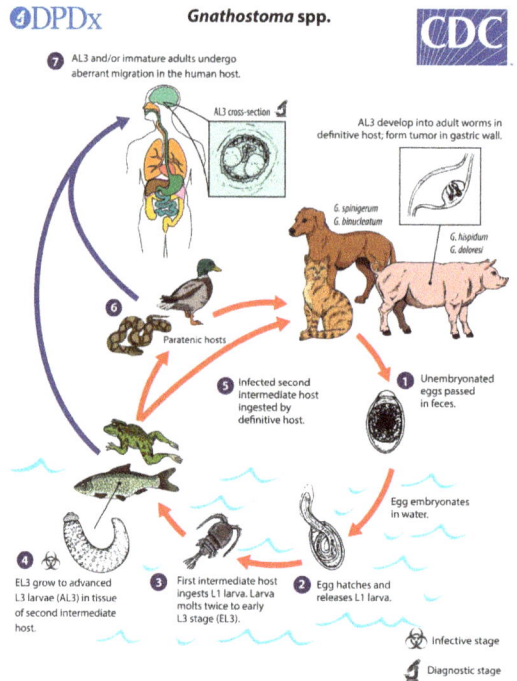

Figure 1. The life cycle of *Gnathostoma* species. (Source: Centers for Disease Control and Prevention, www.dpd.cdc.gov/dpdx/gnathostomiasis/index.html). The adult nematodes occupy the stomach of definitive host animals in the form of a tumour-like mass, and their eggs are passed out in faeces. In water the egg hatches to release a free-swimming ensheathed larva, which after being eaten by the first intermediate host, a small copepod (e.g., *Cyclops* sp.), progresses to the second stage (L2 larva) and early third-stage larva (L3) in its haemocoel. When the infected copepod is ingested by a second intermediate host (usually a fish, of various species, but also crustaceans, eels, frogs, snakes, birds, or mammals), the L3 larva migrates to muscle, and encysts. The late L3 larva traverses the food chain, through predation of paratenic (transport) hosts on one another. In the definitive (final) host, the larva migrates to the stomach via the abdominal cavity and liver, and matures into the adult nematode within about 6 to 12 months. Humans are typically infected when they eat raw or undercooked fish or other intermediate hosts, including eels and crabs; proposed alternative routes of infection are swallowing water containing infected copepods, and direct invasion by L3 larvae through the skin of people handling raw fish or meat [4,5].

This report describes two patients with laboratory-confirmed gnathostomiasis related to raw fish consumption in the Okavango River delta, and a cluster of probable cases with a similar exposure history and suggestive clinical features. The Okavango delta is a unique inland aquatic ecosystem located in northeast Botswana (Figure 2) that attracts many tourists, some of whom are from southern African countries. The purpose of this report is to place these cases of gnathostomiasis on record, and to alert visitors, local residents, and tourism operators to this emerging, potentially serious health risk that is fortunately readily avoidable.

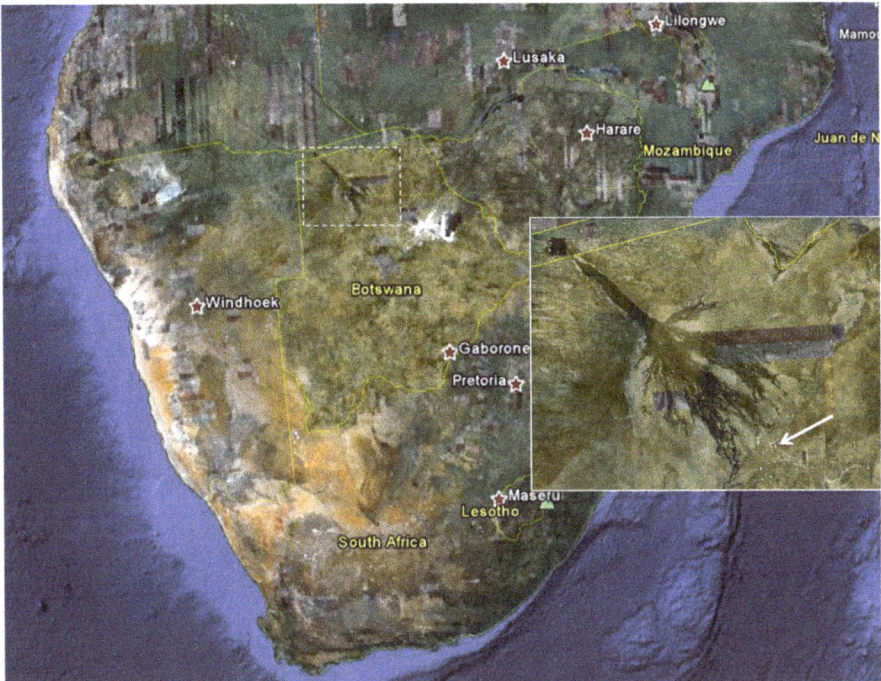

Figure 2. Satellite image of southern Africa. Dashed outline: Okavango delta region in northeast Botswana. Inset: Enlarged view of Okavango delta region showing location of Maun (arrow). (Source: Google Maps, www.google.com/maps/).

Ethical clearance: All investigation and publication of cases or outbreaks of communicable diseases is carried out by the National Institute for Communicable Diseases under ethical clearance from the Human Research Ethics Committee (Medical) of the University of the Witwatersrand, clearance certificate no. M160667.

2. Case Descriptions

2.1. Cases 1 and 2

The patients were a middle-aged married expatriate couple living in Maun, Botswana (Figure 2, inset). Both had experienced several episodes of recurrent painful skin nodules (Figure 3A), associated with transient urticarial reactions. The most recent episode had occurred within a few weeks of a trip to the Okavango delta, where (as they usually did on such trips) they had eaten fillets of raw bream (the common name for several indigenous fish species belonging to the family Cichlidae, e.g., *Sargochromis giardi*, *Serrochromis robustus*, and *Coptodon rendalli*) that had been marinated in lemon juice. On this occasion the husband also complained of nonspecific malaise, and the wife developed a painful migratory skin lesion on her left breast (Figure 3B). Some of the nodular skin lesions were superficial, and from several of them, the patients were able to manually express small worms, about 6–10 mm long (Figure 4A). Due to his systemic symptoms, the husband consulted a medical practitioner. Laboratory investigations revealed a haemoglobin level and leucocyte count (16.1 g/dL and 7.5×10^9/L, respectively) within normal ranges, but a high absolute eosinophilia of 1.69×10^9/L (upper limit of normal range is 0.45×10^9/L). Neither the erythrocyte sedimentation rate nor the c-reactive protein level was elevated. One of the worms removed from the skin was preserved in 40% ethanol and sent to the Parasitology Reference Laboratory at the National Institute for Communicable Diseases in

Johannesburg, South Africa. Microscopic examination revealed the typical morphological features of the L3 larval stage of a *Gnathostoma* species (Figure 4B,C,D).

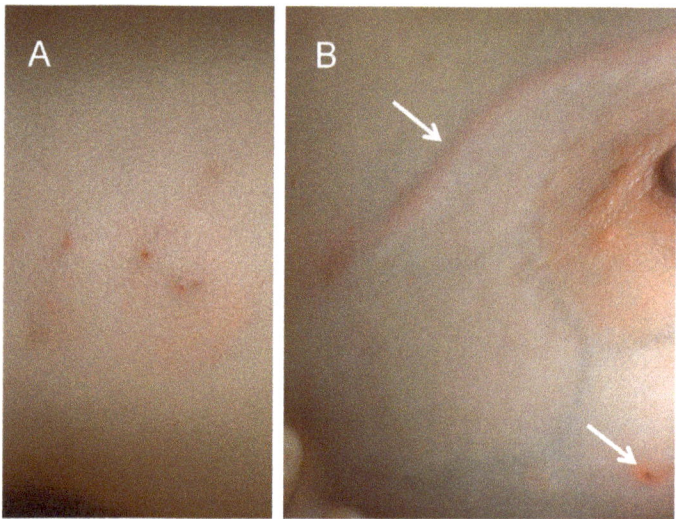

Figure 3. (**A**) Skin nodules caused by localised *Gnathostoma* sp. L3 larvae. (**B**) Linear larva migrans lesion on skin of breast (upper arrow) and skin nodule (lower arrow).

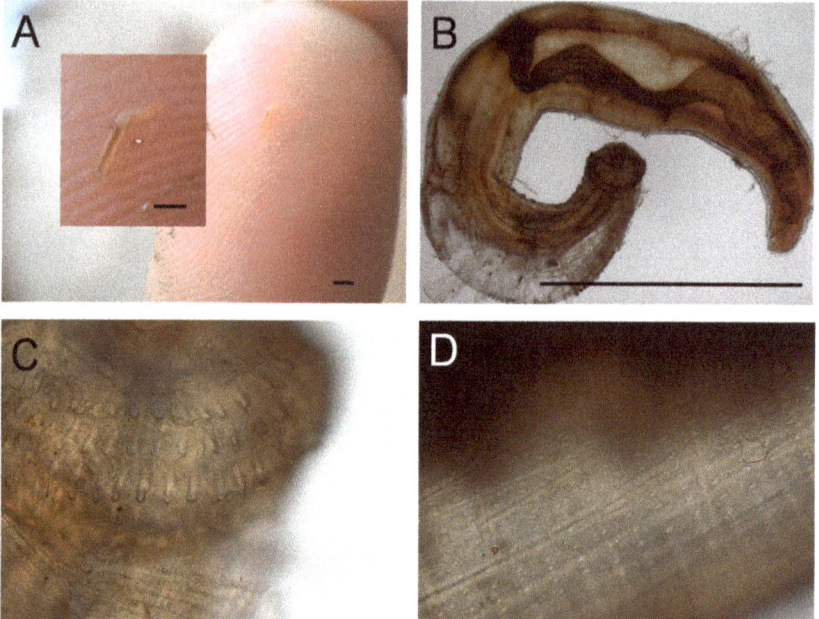

Figure 4. *Gnathostoma* sp. L3 larva. (**A**) As extracted from skin lesion. (**B**) View under ×4 objective. (**C**) Head showing four rows of hooks, ×10 objective. (**D**) Body showing rows of spines, ×10 objective. Bars are approx. 2 mm.

2.2. Cases 3–5

An outbreak of probable gnathostomiasis occurred among staff and passengers who had been aboard a houseboat that was cruising in the Okavango delta, although laboratory confirmation of these cases is lacking. Four persons on the boat ate freshly-caught raw bream, marinated in lemon juice. Three of the four developed symptoms and signs of gnathostomiasis, including painful migratory subcutaneous lesions. Detailed clinical features are only known for one adult male patient who, five days after eating the raw fish, developed severe diarrhoea and vomiting, followed by headaches and mild fever. Laboratory investigations for malaria and schistosomiasis were negative, and the full blood count and liver function tests were normal. The headaches, fever, and fatigue persisted for more than a week. Eleven days after onset of symptoms, the patient developed severe pain in his right flank and right axilla, spreading posteriorly to the scapula area, suggesting a migratory inflammatory process. On the basis of the geographical, dietary and clinical history, and knowledge of published descriptions of cases acquired in the same area, a clinical diagnosis of gnathostomiasis was made and empiric treatment with albendazole (400 mg daily) was started. Pain and headaches subsided quite quickly, but fatigue persisted until almost the end of the 21-day treatment period. Two other patients with the same symptoms, who respectively received ivermectin and albendazole, also recovered well.

3. Discussion

Humans are sometimes accidentally infected with *Gnathostoma* species, which are nematode parasites of fish-eating animals, usually wild and domestic cats and dogs, but the host range of this parasite genus extends to pigs, rodents, raccoons, opossums, otters, weasels and other mustelids, and bears. Among 13 recognised species worldwide, there are at least six that infect humans, the most common of which is *Gnathostoma spinigerum* (reviewed in [1,3]). The species are traditionally differentiated on morphological features, but modern nucleic acid-based methods have also been utilised.

Gnathostomiasis is well known in southeast Asian countries, especially Thailand; the geographic extent includes India, Bangladesh, China, Korea, Japan, and Central and South America (particularly Mexico, Peru, and Equador, countries where ceviche, raw fish marinated in lime juice, is popular) [3,6–8]. Africa is a relatively recently recognised risk region for the disease. Three cases from the Rufiji River in southeastern Tanzania have been described (cited in [9]). A man who had lived in South Africa and who presented with eosinophilic oesophagitis, had a positive serological test for *G. spinigerum*, but he had also lived in Southeast Asia, where the disease is common [10]. Previous small outbreaks of gnathostomiasis acquired in the Okavango and nearby western Zambia region have been reported [9,11], but none of these involved South Africans. Captive lions in Namibia and Zimbabwe had eggs of *Gnathostoma* species detected in their faeces by microscopy, additional evidence of endemicity of the parasite in the region [12,13]. The disease is probably more common in humans in southern Africa than is realised, being relatively or completely unknown and therefore not recognised locally; also, laboratory diagnosis is not readily available. The regional epidemiology of human and animal gnathostomiasis, particularly whether the disease affects local inhabitants of the Okavango region, along with surveys of potential intermediate hosts, clearly requires scientific investigation. The southern African cases all acquired the infection by eating raw bream that had been marinated in lemon juice (that is, a version of ceviche), which, according to the patients, is a popular delicacy provided to tourists visiting the delta, suggesting that the risk of acquiring gnathostomiasis continues to exist.

The L3 larvae, measuring up to 12.5 mm in length by 1.2 mm in width, typically migrate through skin and subcutaneous tissues producing painful migratory swellings (the most common presentation). As in the first cases described above, the presentation may be of cutaneous larva migrans (creeping eruption), or localised skin nodules from which the larvae may emerge or be removed. Sometimes larvae invade internal organs including pulmonary, gastrointestinal, or genitourinary systems, or occasionally, the eyes and central nervous system in the most serious forms of the disease. The range of central nervous system disease includes eosinophilic meningitis or meningoencephalitis, radiculomyelitis/encephalitis, and subarachnoid haemorrhage, and may be fatal in up to 25% of cases (reviewed in [7]). Without treatment, the larvae may live for more than ten years. The pathogenesis of gnathostomiasis is related to the mechanical tissue damage produced by the rapid active movement of the migrating larvae, the various secretions and excretions they produce, and the host immune response. Haemorrhagic tracks in the subcutaneous tissue and internal organs typically mark the passage of the larvae [4,7].

Regarding the differential diagnosis, there are several other fish-borne nematode parasites of humans, namely *Anisakis* spp., *Pseudoterranova* spp., *Capillaria philippinensis*, and some other nematode species that very rarely cause disease in humans. However, the clinical presentation of these infections is predominantly gastrointestinal symptoms, unlike gnathostomiasis. Sparganosis, a metacestode disease acquired from raw fish, can also produce soft tissue swellings that are sometimes migratory, but is much slower than gnathostomiasis to develop, requiring years or decades to become clinically evident.

In endemic areas, the diagnosis of gnathostomiasis is usually made by the combination of clinical features and history of consuming undercooked aquatic food items, or sometimes, unusual risk items such as raw snake meat or live fish [1,14]. The rdiagnosis is supported by the finding of eosinophilia in blood (or cerebrospinal fluid, in the case of central nervous system involvement); however, eosinophilia is not invariable, as in our probable case where the differential leucocyte count was normal. In a British case series of gnathostomiasis in travellers, eight of 16 patients had normal eosinophil counts [11]. Various serological tests have been used, some of which have crossreacted with antibodies against other nematodes. Currently, the preferred laboratory test is immunoblotdetection of a specific 24-kDa antigen produced by *G. spinigerum* L3 larvae, but availability of this investigation is limited to certain tropical disease laboratories in Thailand and Switzerland [7,9].

Effective treatment (albendazole, 400 mg BD for 21 days) for cutaneous infection is available in South Africa. Ivermectin (0.2 mg/kg as a single dose, or 0.2 mg/kg on two consecutive days) is also a suitable anthelminthic drug, but is not routinely available in South Africa. Repeat treatment is sometimes necessary [8]. A sudden rise in absolute eosinophil count may indicate treatment failure. Treating central nervous system invasion is more difficult and corticosteroids might be advisable to reduce the inflammatory response to the parasite [15], but a clinical trial showed no benefit from steroid treatment. In the limited southern African experience of gnathostomiasis to date, there have been no apparent cases of visceral, central nervous system, or ocular involvement.

4. Conclusions

Imported gnathostomiasis is an emerging disease resulting from increasing international travel and adventurous eating. Encysted gnathostome larvae in fish are not killed by marinating in lemon or lime juice, salting, or sun-drying. Tourists and recreational fishermen in the Okavango region, as well as other southern African destinations, are advised not to eat raw locally-caught freshwater fish, and tour operators should educate their local guides not to offer this delicacy to tourists.

Funding: This research received no external funding.

Acknowledgments: The author thanks Chris Carey, Maun, Botswana, for assistance in obtaining case information.

Conflicts of Interest: The author declares no conflict of interest.

References

1. Eiras, J.C.; Pavanelli, G.C.; Takemoto, R.M.; Nawa, Y. An Overview of Fish-borne Nematodiases among Returned Travelers for Recent 25 Years—Unexpected Diseases Sometimes Far Away from the Origin. *Korean J. Parasitol.* **2018**, *56*, 215–227. [CrossRef] [PubMed]
2. Cole, R.A.; Choudhury, A.; Nico, L.G.; Griffin, K.M. *Gnathostoma spinigerum* in live Asian swamp eels (*Monopterus* spp.) from food markets and wild populations, United States. *Emerg. Infect. Dis.* **2014**, *20*, 634–642. [CrossRef] [PubMed]

3. Diaz, J.H. Gnathostomiasis: An Emerging Infection of Raw Fish Consumers in *Gnathostoma* Nematode-Endemic and Nonendemic Countries. *J. Travel Med.* **2015**, *22*, 318–324. [CrossRef] [PubMed]
4. Miyazaki, I. *An Illustrated Book of Helminthic Zoonoses*; International Medical Foundation of Japan: Tokyo, Japan, 1991; pp. 368–409.
5. Daengsvang, S. Human gnathostomiasis in Siam with reference to the method of prevention. *J. Parasitol.* **1949**, *35*, 116–121. [CrossRef] [PubMed]
6. Eiras, J.C.; Pavanelli, G.C.; Takemoto, R.M.; Nawa, Y. Fish-borne nematodiases in South America: Neglected emerging diseases. *J. Helminthol.* **2018**, *92*, 649–654. [CrossRef] [PubMed]
7. Herman, J.S.; Chiodini, P.L. Gnathostomiasis, another emerging imported disease. *Clin. Microbiol. Rev.* **2009**, *22*, 484–492. [CrossRef] [PubMed]
8. Moore, D.A.; McCroddan, J.; Dekumyoy, P.; Chiodini, P.L. Gnathostomiasis: An emerging imported disease. *Emerg. Infect. Dis.* **2003**, *9*, 647–650. [CrossRef] [PubMed]
9. Hale, D.C.; Blumberg, L.; Frean, J. Case report: Gnathostomiasis in two travelers to Zambia. *Am. J. Trop. Med. Hyg.* **2003**, *68*, 707–709. [CrossRef] [PubMed]
10. Müller-Stöver, I.; Richter, J.; Häussinger, D. Infection with *Gnathostoma spinigerum* as a cause of eosinophilic oesophagitis. *Dtsch. Med. Wochenschr.* **2004**, *29*, 1973–1975. [CrossRef] [PubMed]
11. Herman, J.S.; Wall, E.C.; van-Tulleken, C.; Godfrey-Faussett, P.; Bailey, R.L.; Chiodini, P.L. Gnathostomiasis acquired by British tourists in Botswana. *Emerg. Infect. Dis.* **2009**, *15*, 594–597. [CrossRef] [PubMed]
12. Mukarati, N.L.; Vassilev, G.D.; Tagwireyi, W.M.; Tavengwa, M. Occurrence, prevalence and intensity of internal parasite infections of African lions (*Panthera leo*) in enclosures at a recreation park in Zimbabwe. *J. Zoo Wildl. Med.* **2013**, *44*, 686–693. [CrossRef] [PubMed]
13. Smith, Y.; Kok, O.B. Faecal helminth egg and oocyst counts of a small population of African lions (*Panthera leo*) in the southwestern Kalahari, Namibia. *Onderstepoort J. Vet. Res.* **2006**, *73*, 71–75. [CrossRef] [PubMed]
14. Nawa, Y.; Hatz, C.; Blum, J. Sushi delights and parasites: The risk of fishborne and foodborne parasitic zoonoses in Asia. *Clin. Infect. Dis.* **2005**, *41*, 1297–1303. [CrossRef] [PubMed]
15. Leroy, J.; Cornu, M.; Deleplancque, A.S.; Loridant, S.; Dutoit, E.; Sendid, B. Sushi, ceviche and gnathostomiasis—A case report and review of imported infections. *Travel Med. Infect. Dis.* **2017**, *20*, 26–30. [CrossRef] [PubMed]

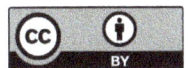

© 2020 by the author. Licensee MDPI, Basel, Switzerland. This article is an open access article distributed under the terms and conditions of the Creative Commons Attribution (CC BY) license (http://creativecommons.org/licenses/by/4.0/).

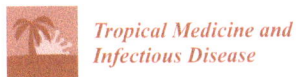

Case Report

Percutaneous Emergence of *Gnathostoma spinigerum* Following Praziquantel Treatment

Sarah G. H. Sapp [1,*], Monica Kaminski [2], Marie Abdallah [2], Henry S. Bishop [1], Mark Fox [1,3], MacKevin Ndubuisi [1] and Richard S. Bradbury [1]

1. Parasitic Diseases Branch, Division of Parasitic Diseases and Malaria, Center for Global Health, Centers for Disease Control and Prevention, Atlanta, GA 30029, USA; hsb2@cdc.gov (H.S.B.); nyg3@cdc.gov (M.F.); nrm6@cdc.gov (M.N.); rbradbur76@gmail.com (R.S.B.)
2. New York City Health and Hospitals Corporation, New York, NY 10013, USA; Monica.Kaminski@downstate.edu (M.K.); marie.abdallah@nychhc.org (M.A.)
3. Oak Ridge Institute for Science and Education, Oak Ridge Associated Universities, Oak Ridge, TN 37830, USA
* Correspondence: xyz6@cdc.gov

Received: 4 November 2019; Accepted: 11 December 2019; Published: 14 December 2019

Abstract: A Bangladeshi patient with prior travel to Saudi Arabia was hospitalized in the United States for a presumptive liver abscess. Praziquantel was administered following a positive *Schistosoma* antibody test. Ten days later, a subadult worm migrated to the skin surface and was identified morphologically as *Gnathostoma spinigerum*. This case highlights the challenges of gnathostomiasis diagnosis, raising questions on potential serologic cross-reactivity and the possible role of praziquantel in stimulating outward migration of *Gnathostoma* larvae/subadults.

Keywords: gnathostomiasis; schistosomiasis; imported helminthiasis; praziquantel

1. Introduction

Gnathostomiasis is a foodborne zoonosis with diverse and sometimes serious clinical outcomes. Transmission occurs via consumption of advanced third-stage (AL3) larvae encysted in undercooked meat of intermediate or paratenic hosts, commonly freshwater fish, frogs, snakes, and fowl. Larvae undergo an invasive course of migration in the aberrant human host after penetrating the gastrointestinal wall, first migrating to the liver parenchyma and then other organs [1]. The usual presentation is cutaneous gnathostomiasis, frequently preceded by a nonspecific prodrome due to larval migration. Other presentations include urogenital, visceral, ocular, and neurological gnathostomiasis [1,2]. Management can be challenging with frequent relapses or treatment failures [3].

The known zoonotic species are *Gnathostoma spinigerum*, *G. hispidum*, *G. doloresi*, *G. nipponicum*, *G. binucleatum*, and possibly *G. malaysiae* [1,2]. Among these, *G. spinigerum* is the best-studied with the broadest occurrence; this species is endemic across Southeast Asia, East Asia, India, Africa, and possibly Australia [1]. Gnathostomiasis has been recognized as a parasitic infection of travelers and refugees from endemic regions [2,4], however, awareness among general practitioners in nonendemic countries may be limited.

2. Case Report

In June 2018, a 46-year-old female originally from Bangladesh (emigrated to the USA in 2017) presented to her primary care physician with complaints of diarrhea. The patient had traveled to Saudi Arabia for ten days and developed symptoms one week after returning to the USA. She was prescribed a 7-day course of metronidazole, though she only complied for 2 days due to religious fasting. Two weeks following symptom onset, the patient was admitted to the hospital with diffuse intermittent abdominal pain that began two days earlier and continuing diarrhea. She reported epigastric and right upper abdominal quadrant (RUQ) pain and increased belching. No other signs/symptoms were reported or observed.

Upon admission she was afebrile and had stable vital signs. Physical examination revealed mild discomfort to deep palpation of the epigastrium and RUQ. Her white blood cell (WBC) count was elevated at 20.64×10^9/L (normal $(4.70–10.30) \times 10^9$/L) with 57.8% eosinophils, 18.8% neutrophils, 19.7% lymphocytes, and 0.5% basophils. A CT scan of the abdomen showed diffuse gastric wall thickening with mild adjacent inflammatory change, suggestive of gastritis, and a hypodensity in the left lower liver measuring 2.2 cm with a rim enhancing wall, suspicious for abscess. Metronidazole and ceftriaxone treatment was initiated. Interventional radiology was consulted for liver abscess drainage, but the procedure was deferred in view of the small size. The abdominal pain resolved on the second day of hospitalization, but the patient remained admitted for continuation of IV antibiotic treatment.

On the third day of hospitalization, serum and stool specimens were collected and sent for testing for various parasitic etiologies, including schistosomiasis, to determine the cause of peripheral eosinophilia and liver abscess. Antibody tests for *Entamoeba histolytica*, *Strongyloides*, and *Toxocara* and a pan-filarial assay were negative. Three of four stool examinations were negative (one positive for *Blastocystis*). The patient was discharged on day 8 following placement of a peripherally-inserted central catheter for the continuation of intravenous ceftriaxone (6-week course) and oral metronidazole for liver abscess treatment.

Five weeks following discharge, a RUQ sonogram showed abscess resolution, however, blood work revealed persistent WBC elevation (17.66×10^9/L) with 46.1% eosinophils, 29.0% neutrophils, 20.6% lymphocytes, 2.9% monocytes, and 0.5% basophils. She was advised to continue ceftriaxone/metronidazole for another week. A few days later, a low positive result was returned for the previously-ordered *Schistosoma* antibody test (FAST-ELISA value 13.0 (0–10 normal)); ceftriaxone/metronidazole was ceased and praziquantel (40 mg/kg in 2 doses taken in one day) was prescribed. Ten days after praziquantel treatment, the patient reported epigastric pain with localized rash, pruritus, and hyperesthesia. Clinical examination identified a serpiginous track with an emerging worm over the upper abdomen (Figure 1) which was extracted. Photos of the parasite were submitted for telediagnosis to the Centers for Disease Control and Prevention (Atlanta, Georgia, USA). The specimen was stored in 70% ethanol and shipped for morphologic examination.

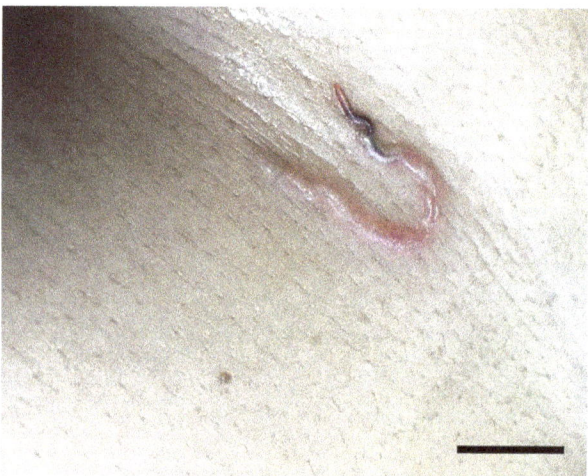

Figure 1. Serpiginous track showing the emerging subcutaneous *Gnathostoma spinigerum*. (Bar = approximately 1 cm).

By microscopy, the gross appearance and the presence of a cephalic bulb and broad caudal alae (Figure 2) were characteristic of a subadult male *Gnathostoma*. The total length was 0.66 cm; other morphometric characteristics are summarized in Table 1. The cephalic bulb had two lips and cephalic spines were simple, arranged in eight alternating rows. The blunt posterior was difficult to assess in detail due to the position in which the worm was fixed; caudal alae were broad and rounded. The extremities were deep red in color, and body spines began after the cephalic bulb. Anterior spines were mostly tricuspidate, occasionally quadricuspidate, with points of roughly even length. Further posteriad, spines became elongate and bicuspidate and eventually became single points before an aspinous area at ~60% of the distance from the anterior. Sparse, simple spines were present on the interior portion of caudal alae (Figure 2).

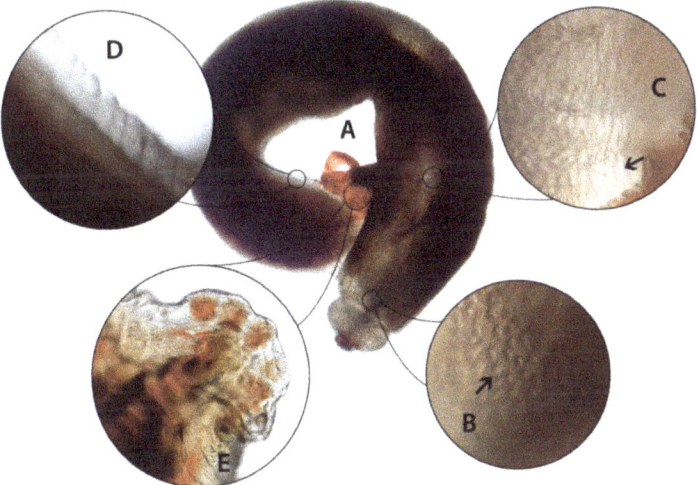

Figure 2. Subadult male *Gnathostoma spinigerum* extracted from the patient. (**A**) Whole worm, measuring 0.66 cm; (**B**) short, three-pointed spines just behind cephalic bulb; (**C**) longer spines on anterior half of body; (**D**) aspinous area of the posterior body; (**E**) caudal alae showing round pedunculate papillae and surface texture with simple spines. Photos of spines taken under 200× magnification.

Table 1. Morphometric characteristics of the subadult *Gnathostoma spinigerum* male extracted from the patient.

Aspect	Size
Total length	0.66 cm
Cephalic bulb maximal width	575 μm
Cephalic bulb length	300 μm
Width immediately behind cephalic bulb	675 μm
Width at midbody	950 μm
Width before posterior	700 μm
Caudal alae	260 μm widest 210 μm narrowest

Based on detailed microscopic examination and characteristics of the body spines, this worm was identified as *Gnathostoma spinigerum*. The shape and distribution of spines were sufficient to rule out other zoonotic *Gnathostoma* spp. using published descriptions. PCR was also attempted on a small fragment of the worm, but insufficient DNA was extracted and amplification was unsuccessful. The patient was treated with ivermectin (0.2 mg/kg, 2 days) following confirmation of the diagnosis, resulting in resolution of symptoms and eosinophilia. A follow-up abdominal CT scan one month later was normal.

3. Discussion

We identified an imported case of cutaneous gnathostomiasis caused by a subadult male *G. spinigerum* with some interesting characteristics. *Gnathostoma* spp. diagnosed in cases of deeper tissue involvement (e.g. brain, urogenital, liver) are typically of a larval stage, but worms from cutaneous cases may show a variable degree of maturation, although never reaching sexual maturity [2,5]. Recovery of the intact, subadult worm allowed for species determination based on body spines, which is more straightforward than on advanced third-stage larvae (AL3). For example, all but one zoonotic *Gnathostoma* species have AL3 with four rows of cephalic hooklets, and body spines are not sufficiently developed [1,5]. Histological sectioning allows examination of intestinal cell morphology, but this may be difficult to distinguish except in ideal lateral sections [6].

Spontaneous percutaneous emergence is relatively rare in gnathostomiasis cases; however, this may apparently be induced by drug treatment. Albendazole was demonstrated to stimulate outward migration of *G. spinigerum* larvae in a clinical trial involving Thai patients presenting with serologically-confirmed cutaneous gnathostomiasis [7]. Emergence did not occur among 40 patients in the placebo-treated group but was recorded three times in the group receiving albendazole (400 mg, 2× daily for 12 days). These events occurred 8–14 days following treatment and were preceded by erythematous linear or papular lesions on areas where worms eventually emerged. In two patients, the larvae were superficial enough that they were removed by squeezing or with a needle [7]. Percutaneous emergence has also been noted sporadically following single-dose ivermectin treatment (0.2 mg/kg), though more detailed clinical information is unavailable [8,9]. The development of migratory, swollen nodules was also reported in association with interferon alpha-2b injections for hepatitis C, although in this patient the worm did not emerge percutaneously until after nine months of therapy [10]. While additional targeted studies will be necessary to definitively implicate praziquantel as a larval migratory stimulus, the emergence of the worm in this patient mirrors the presentation and timing observed in the albendazole trial, suggesting that the emergence could possibly have been stimulated by the drug. The mechanism by which outward migration is stimulated is not known, including whether it represents directional or random motility; it is also not clear why a drug with no appreciable nematocidal activity would induce emergence. The nematode cuticle is believed to confer resistance to the calcium-channel-disrupting effects observed in Platyhelminthes, but nematodes may still uptake small amounts of praziquantel orally [11,12].

As some cases of gnathostomiasis have also been initially misdiagnosed as schistosomiasis [13,14], it is important that clinicians consider the likelihood of exposure, clinical features, and serologic results in differential diagnosis. However, the overlapping geographic ranges of these parasites, nonspecific clinical manifestations, and difficulty of serologic interpretation present a challenge—particularly if patients report complex travel history. Our patient presented with eosinophilia and was positive for *Schistosoma* antibody, prompting praziquantel treatment. She had recently returned from Saudi Arabia, but the testing was within the five-week minimum period required for seroconversion in schistosomiasis [15,16]. Exposures within a year or two prior were unlikely since Bangladesh is schistosomiasis nonendemic [17]. This raises the possibility that the *G. spinigerum* infection generated antibodies that reacted with the schistosomiasis antigen in the FAST-ELISA. Some schistosomiasis seroassays have known cross-reactivity with nematode infections, and anti-*Gnathostoma* antibodies were shown to cross-react in the *Schistosoma mekongi*-specific SmkAWA ELISA [15]. Similarly to our case, serologic testing for *Schistosoma mansoni* in one reported gnathostomiasis case from Brazil was weakly positive, which lead to an initial incorrect diagnosis of schistosomiasis [14]. The low value of the FAST-ELISA result, lack of follow-up, and negative stool examination suggest that cross-reactivity was likely in our patient's case. Alternately, the low level of *Schistosoma* antibody could possibly indicate a very old infection; it unknown if the patient had visited Saudi Arabia on multiple occasions prior to the reported visit. Overall, these findings highlight the importance of investigating potential serological cross-reactivity created by *Gnathostoma* infections, which may go undetected and mislead treatment decisions. Adding to the diagnostic challenge presented by gnathostomiasis is the very limited availability of serologic testing for *Gnathostoma* spp. (not available in the United States). As far as clinical evidence, gastric wall and liver involvement observed in this patient are more consistent with gnathostomiasis, as migration of *Gnathostoma* larvae involves the stomach penetration and liver parenchyma invasion and long latent periods (months to years) can occur, supporting the notion that the *G. spinigerum* was acquired some time ago in the endemic region [1,3,6].

Further research is necessary to understand the relationship between *Gnathostoma* emergence and praziquantel. Drug-induced stimulation of worm migration presents a hypothetical risk if such stimulation represents an increase in random migration. Larvae could perhaps invade deeper tissues rather than emerging through skin, with more dire clinical outcomes. Clinicians should be aware of the possibility of "uncovering" latent *Gnathostoma* infections following anthelmintic treatment in patients from endemic regions.

Author Contributions: S.G.H.S. and M.K. wrote manuscript; S.G.H.S., H.S.B., M.N., M.F., and R.S.B. performed specimen intake, examination, and interpretation; M.A. and M.K. managed patient and provided clinical history.

Funding: This research received no external funding.

Acknowledgments: We would like to thank John Quale (New York City Health and Hospitals Corporation) for specimen submission and coordinating communication between laboratories. The patient in this case report provided written informed consent for publication (CDC Division of Parasitic Diseases and Malaria human subjects project ID 0900f3eb81932f08).

Conflicts of Interest: The authors declare no conflict of interest.

Disclaimer: The findings and conclusions in this report are those of the authors and do not necessarily represent the official position of the Centers for Disease Control and Prevention.

References

1. Miyazaki, I. *An Illustrated Book of Helminthic Zoonoses*; International Medical Foundation of Japan: Tokyo, Japan, 1991.
2. Waikagul, J.; Chamacho, S.D. Gnathostomiasis. In *Food-Borne Parasitic Zoonoses*; Springer: New York, NY, USA, 2007; pp. 235–261.
3. Strady, C.; Dekumyoy, P.; Clement-Rigolet, M.; Danis, M.; Bricaire, F.; Caumes, E. Long-term follow-up of imported gnathostomiasis shows frequent treatment failure. *Am. J. Trop. Med. Hyg.* **2009**, *80*, 33–35. [CrossRef] [PubMed]
4. Herman, J.S.; Chiodini, P.L. Gnathostomiasis, another emerging imported disease. *Clin. Microbiol. Rev.* **2009**, *22*, 484–492. [CrossRef] [PubMed]
5. Radomyos, P.; Daengsvang, S. A brief report on *Gnathostoma spinigerum* specimens obtained from human cases. *Southeast Asian J. Trop. Med. Public Health* **1987**, *18*, 215–217. [PubMed]
6. Miyazaki, I. On the genus *Gnathostoma* and human gnathostomiasis, with special reference to Japan. *Exp. Parasitol.* **1960**, *9*, 338–370. [CrossRef]
7. Suntharasamai, P.; Riganti, M.; Chittamas, S.; Desakorn, V. Albendazole stimulates outward migration of *Gnathostoma spinigerum* to the dermis in man. *Southeast Asian J. Trop. Med. Public Health* **1992**, *23*, 716–722. [PubMed]
8. Kraivichian, K.; Nuchprayoon, S.; Sitichalernchai, P.; Chaicumpa, W.; Yentakam, S. Treatment of cutaneous gnathostomiasis with ivermectin. *Am. J. Trop. Med. Hyg.* **2004**, *71*, 623–628. [CrossRef] [PubMed]
9. Nontasut, P.; Bussaratid, V.; Chullawichit, S.; Charoensook, N.; Visetsuk, K. Comparison of ivermectin and albendazole treatment for gnathostomiasis. *Southeast Asian J. Trop. Med. Public Health* **2000**, *31*, 374–377. [PubMed]
10. Sangchan, A.; Sawanyawisuth, K.; Intapan, P.M.; Mahakkanukrauh, A. Outward migration of *Gnathostoma spinigerum* in interferon alpha treated Hepatitis C patient. *Parasitol. Int.* **2006**, *55*, 31–32. [CrossRef] [PubMed]
11. Harnett, W. The anthelmintic action of praziquantel. *Parasitol. Today* **1988**, *4*, 144–146. [CrossRef]

12. Andrews, P.; Thomas, H.; Weber, H. The in vitro uptake of 14c-praziquantel by cestodes, trematodes, and a nematode. *J. Parasitol.* **1980**, *66*, 920–925. [CrossRef] [PubMed]
13. Hale, D.C.; Blumberg, L.; Frean, J. Case report: Gnathostomiasis in two travelers to zambia. *Am. J. Trop. Med. Hyg.* **2003**, *68*, 707–709. [CrossRef] [PubMed]
14. de Sousa Vargas, T.J.; Kahler, S.; Dib, C.; Cavaliere, M.B.; Jeunon-Sousa, M.A. Autochthonous gnathostomiasis, Brazil. *Emerg. Infect. Dis.* **2012**, *18*, 2087. [CrossRef] [PubMed]
15. Hinz, R.; Schwarz, N.G.; Hahn, A.; Frickmann, H.J.M. Serological approaches for the diagnosis of schistosomiasis–a review. *Mol. Cell. Probes* **2017**, *31*, 2–21. [CrossRef] [PubMed]
16. Colley, D.G.; Bustinduy, A.L.; Secor, W.E.; King, C.H. Human schistosomiasis. *Lancet* **2014**, *383*, 2253–2264. [CrossRef]
17. World Health Organization. *Schistosomiasis: Status of Schistosomiasis Endemic Countries*; World Health Organization: Geneva, Switzerland, 2017. Available online: https://www.who.int/gho/neglected_diseases/schistosomiasis/en/ (accessed on 1 June 2019).

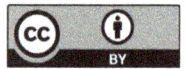

© 2019 by the authors. Licensee MDPI, Basel, Switzerland. This article is an open access article distributed under the terms and conditions of the Creative Commons Attribution (CC BY) license (http://creativecommons.org/licenses/by/4.0/).

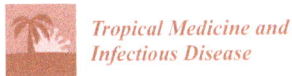 *Tropical Medicine and Infectious Disease*

Brief Report

e-Diagnosis in Medical Parasitology

Harsha Sheorey

Medical Microbiologist, St Vincent's Hospital, Melbourne 3065, Australia; harsha.sheorey@svha.org.au

Received: 19 December 2019; Accepted: 1 January 2020; Published: 3 January 2020

Abstract: Over the past decade or two, the teaching of laboratory diagnostic parasitology has been neglected in Australasia, as parasitic infections are relatively uncommon. As a consequence, expertise in medical parasitology is dwindling. A team of international experts (including Professor John Goldsmid) has been formed to help in the diagnosis of human parasitic infections. The team includes experts from Australia, Europe, South Africa and the USA. Some senior members of the team are excellent morphologists, and we have both human and veterinary parasitologists who help with molecular diagnosis in difficult cases.

Keywords: e-Diagnosis; morphologist; molecular parasitology

Professor John Goldsmid has been a doyen of medical parasitology in Australia for many years. I was honored to meet John during our inaugural parasitology master class organized by the Australian Society for Microbiology (ASM) in Hobart in 2009 (Figure 1). Goldsmid's knowledge, dedication and teaching in this field must be carried on for the future generations of health professionals. His attitude towards learning is exemplary (see response to Case 4 below).

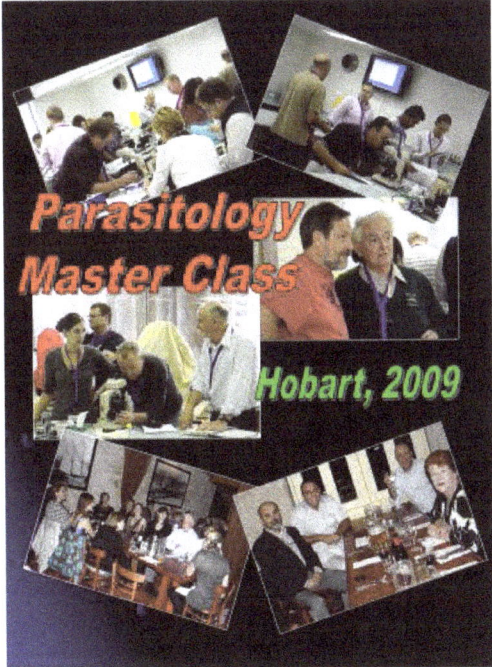

Figure 1. The inaugural Australian parasitology master class.

Over the past decade or two, the teaching of laboratory diagnostic parasitology has been neglected in Australasia because parasitic infections are relatively uncommon. As a consequence, the expertise in medical parasitology is dwindling. While on a sabbatical at the Centre for Disease Control and Prevention in Atlanta (CDC), USA, I came across a method of diagnosing parasites that the parasitology department there had adopted to help less experienced health professionals. A picture of an unknown malarial parasite from Africa was sent to the parasitologists on a smart phone, and, after looking at the image, they were able to send back a diagnosis of malarial parasite to a species level. This method could easily be adopted in Australia, I thought. Thus, a team of experts who have helped in diagnosing and managing parasitic infections was put together.

1. Why e-Diagnosis?

- Less importance/attention is given to parasitic diseases in humans in the developed world (including Australia).
- The re-distribution of parasites due to human/animal movement and environmental and practice changes has brought parasites into the developed world.
- There are declining numbers of experts in this field, especially morphologists.
- The internet 'savvy' public who 'self-diagnose' want to 'confirm' their thoughts.

2. Who Is the Team?

The team includes parasitologists and other experts from Australia, Europe, South Africa, and the USA. Some senior members of the team are excellent morphologists, and we have both human and veterinary parasitologists who help with molecular diagnosis (Figure 2). The author acts as a coordinator of the group. The team has helped diagnose a few unusual parasites, leading to publications [1–4].

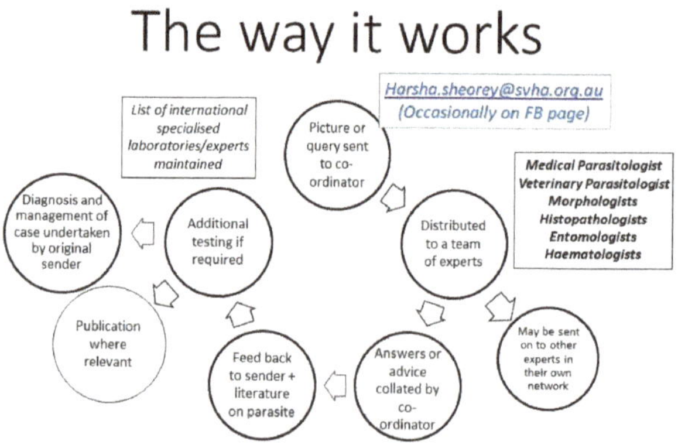

Figure 2. The way e-Diagnosis works.

3. What Kind of Material/Advice is Sought?

Material:

- Images for identification (macroscopic and microscopic)
- Histology sections of tissues with possible parasites

Advice:

- Molecular identification/availability
- Interpretation/availability of serology for parasites

Trop. Med. Infect. Dis. **2020**, *5*, 8

- Advice on testing to exclude parasites
- Management of parasitic infections (treatment and follow-up)—OzBug (Australian email group of interested clinical experts)
- Advice on/to "internet-savvy" patient concerns

4. Type of Parasites Received from Intestine, Tissues or Blood

- Protozoa
- Nematodes
- Trematodes
- Cestodes
- Arthropods
- Pseudo-parasites and artefacts

5. Cases

5.1. Case 1: Lump in the Back (Melbourne, VIC, Australia)

A lump in the back (right scapular region) (Figure 3A) in a young women was biopsied to rule out sarcoma. Its histology showed a helminth with morphological features suggestive of a filarial worm—*Onchocerca* or *Dirofilaria* species (Figure 3B). This prompted the aid of an infectious diseases consult, and history-taking revealed that the patient was a veterinarian with extensive exposure to various animals both in Australia and Africa. Apart from swelling, the patient felt 'movement' inside their nodule. A lumpectomy was performed, and, in the laboratory, the worm fell out of the lump (Figure 3C). On examination, this was confirmed to be a filarial worm with features of *Onchocerca* species (cuticular rings and subcuticular striae) (Figure 3D), most likely a zoonotic *Onchocerca lupi* or *Onchocerca volvulus*.

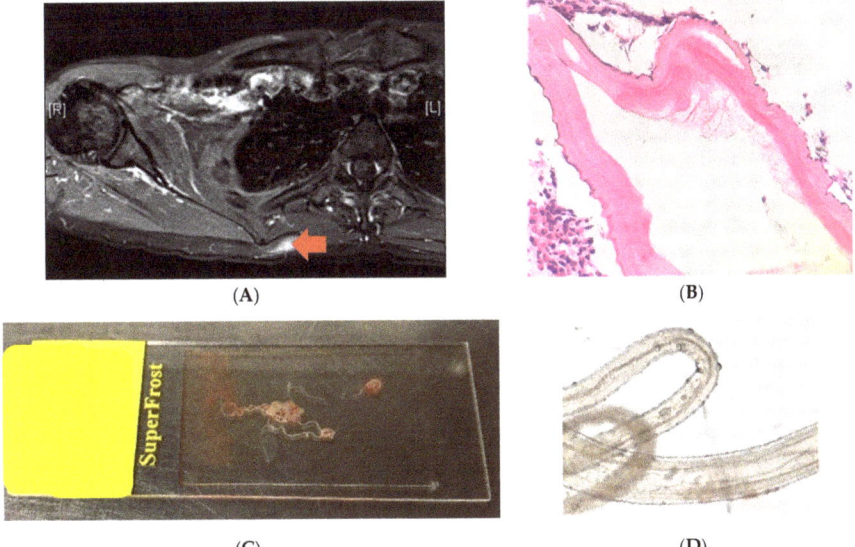

Figure 3. (**A**) PET/CT scan of back showing a lump in the back (red arrow). (**B**) Histology section of the biopsy showing a nematode helminth with features of a filarial worm. (**C**) Intertwined worm(s) fell out of the surgically removed lump. (**D**) On exam, these were found to be two, a thicker female and a thinner male.

e-Diagnosis members views:

Initial histology: Experts were convinced the section had features of a filarial helminth (ridges and internal structures), most likely a zoonotic *Onchocerca* species or *Dirofilaria* species.

After the worm was extracted, experts were convinced that the morphology was most consistent with *Onchocerca* species. A PCR-based sequencing method confirmed it to be *O. volvulus* (1).

5.2. Case 2: Lump in the Axilla (Brisbane, QLD, Australia)

A 23 year old from Brisbane, Australia, presented with an axillary mass for six months. He noticed movement within, and a small worm was expressed. This was placed in formalin. The dimensions were 1.2 mm wide by 3.85 mm long (Figure 4). No relevant travel history was noted.

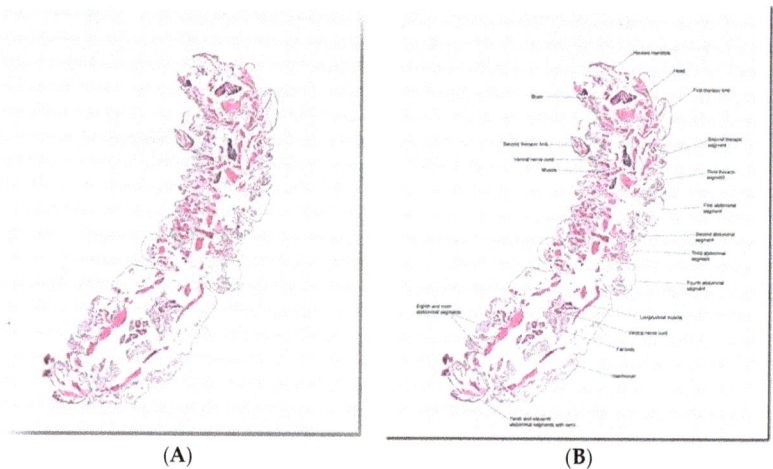

Figure 4. (**A**) Picture of histological section of 'worm' sent to the e-Diagnosis team. (**B**) The same picture that was labelled and sent back to the team by Professor Anderson, showing various morphological features that are consistent with an endopterygota larva.

e-Diagnosis member view:

Professor Emeritus Don Anderson (previously Challis Professor of Zoology at Sydney University)

'An endopterygota larva, most probably a beetle larva with hooked mandibles. A lot of beetle larvae burrow into organic substrates. It's a pity histopathologists almost invariably section things that are more easily identified intact.'

5.3. Case 3: Larvae, Adults and Eggs in CSF/Brain (Adelaide, SA, Australia)

A 73 year old woman was admitted to a regional South Australia hospital (past history with unspecified abdominal pain). The patient was on low dose methotrexate and etanercept for Rheumatoid arthritis (RA). She was transferred to Royal Adelaide Hospital with deteriorating neurological signs. The Cerebro-spinal fluid (CSF) taken showed 280 polymorphs, 18 monocytes, no bacteria seen, high protein, and virology and bacterial PCR and *Cryptococcal* antigen all negative. The CSF taken two days later showed 2500 polymorphs, 34 monocytes, no bacteria seen; Diff-Quik (modified Romanowsky Stain) showed "few eosinophils," and no trophozoites. *Acanthamoeba* cultures were set up. Patient died less than a week after admission, and a post mortem examination was conducted. The CSF at post mortem showed 1700 polymorphs (PMN) (few eosinophils), a very high protein level, and numerous helminth larvae and eggs (Figure 5A,B). *Strongyloides* and *Angiostrongylus* serology was negative. A brain biopsy demonstrated the presence of a helminth. PCR-based sequencing confirmed it to be *Halicephalobus gingivalis* (Figure 5C).

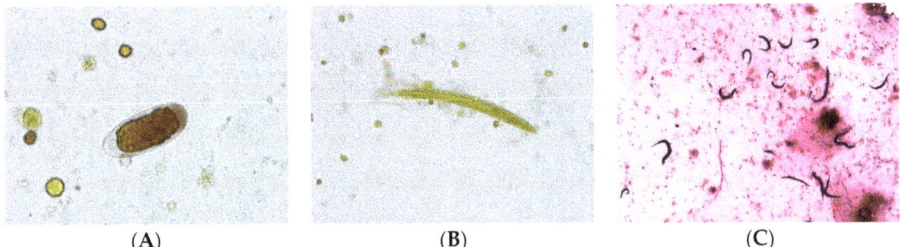

Figure 5. (**A**) Egg of parasite in CSF resembling the *Trichostrongylus* species (~50 × 20 μm). (**B**) larva of parasite in CSF resembling *Strongyloides* species (~250 μm). (**C**) Post-mortem brain tissue showing adult worms, larvae and eggs of the helminth (details and additional pictures in Reference 2).

e-Diagnosis members views:

What follows is a summary of the email discussion that occurred after images were sent to the team. The experts' names are in brackets.

- The structure of the esophagus and ratio to gut may also help us. The two illustrated larvae could just be rhabditiform and hence no notching of tail; there does seem to be a darker region near the genital primordium zone in one photo, but we also lack ability to gain more definition of these key points. (Norbert Ryan).
- The egg looks very much like a *Trichostrongylus* egg (but the size of the eggs is too small), and the larvae have features that are reminiscent of that species also, particularly the wavy pattern of the intestine (John Walker).
- First of all, very few documented cases (of *Strongyloides*) in the brain/CSF. Have no explanation for eggs/rhabditiform larvae in this site (Lynne Garcia).
- I don't think it is the usual suspects, namely *Strongyloides* or *Angiostyrongylus*, on morphological grounds. Eggs are not normally seen in angiostrongyliasis. They look most like stages of *Trichostrongylus*, but that infection does not disseminate, or at least there are no reports thereof. Thus, I think this is a very unusual aberrant infection with *Trichostrongylus* or similar nematode that is not normally found in humans (John Frean).
- I found a lovely description of all stages of *Halicephalobus gingivalis* in Anderson et al. (1998). This is now regarded as the correct name for the parasite. The drawings are very consistent with what is in the images. Note the elongated eggs, the recurved ovaries, and of course the rhabditoid esophagus (Rick Speare).
- Please don't waste the nematodes you have by rushing in and using them immediately for PCR. They should be morphologically described first; then do PCR. Additionally, some should be kept in case it is a new species. Don't forget the light microscopy and measurements, as well as SEM. Of course, the latter looks more spectacular but usually carries less taxonomic weight (Rick Speare).
- The sequence results have come back, and the worms are positive for *Halicephalobus gingivalis*. The 28s D2/D3 primers from Nadler's 2003 paper were used and got the sequence found below (2). This sample was 99% identical to GenBank accession AY294177 over 786 base pairs (Anson Kohler).
- The combination of case details, plus description of the nematodes, plus PCR gives the maximum value. Fabulous effort! Good example of the value of a collaborative dispersed group in diagnosing unusual parasites! (Rick Speare)

5.4. Case 4: Worm Passed in Feces (Wollongong, NSW, Australia)

From Dr. Peter Newton, Pathologist in Wollongong: This worm was sent to us for identification from one of our regional hospitals 80 km away. The history that we received from the ID physician who sent it to us was that of a 75 year old female patient admitted with severe Clostridium difficile-associated disease (CDAD). Her condition has apparently been slowly improving. Yesterday, she was incontinent of feces on the ward floor, and this worm was seen wriggling out of her feces on the floor (Figure 6).

Based on a Google search, we think that it is a "hammerhead worm" of the *Bipalium* genus. We assume it was on the floor and crawled into her feces, or the feces landed on the worm on the floor. It was a rather wet morning on the New South Wales (NSW) coast yesterday, so presumably came onto the ward on someone's shoe. Would value your opinion.

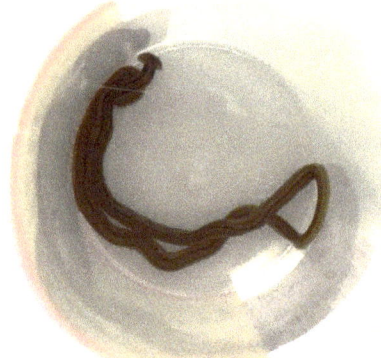

Figure 6. Worm thought to have wriggled out of feces on the floor in an incontinent patient.

e-Diagnosis members view/comments:

Dr. John Walker (ex-Head of Parasitology, Westmead Hospital, Sydney)

The worm is *Bipalium kewense*, first described at Kew Gardens but originally from Southeast Asia. Now has a cosmopolitan distribution as a consequence of trade in botanical specimens. It's a predatory, free-living planarian.

Prof John Goldsmid (UTas, Hobart)

My goodness—we live and learn, even in retirement!! I have never seen this worm or heard of a "hammerhead worm." Peter's tentative identification seems reasonable and probable. I congratulate him on his detective work.

6. Limitations of This Diagnostic Procedure

- Poor images may be sent:
    - Not enough images: multiple images at different magnification levels and that cover key parts of the parasite are not always sent.
    - Poor quality photos that are out of focus or focused on wrong part may be sent. The new smart phones take very good images, so this should not be an excuse.
- No relevant history: Age, epidemiology, travel, exotic food, contact with animals, medication, immune status are all important, and, quite often, this is not communicated.
- Arthropods or large worms received in formalin and sectioned: Arthropods and large worms are better photographed whole and not sectioned. When stored in 70% alcohol, formalin makes specimens 'brittle.'

- 'Degenerate' or dying parasite (histology-section): Morphology may not be typical enough to make a diagnosis.
- Not enough follow up material: The specimen or multiple images should be held onto if required for further identification.
- Direct contact with non-scientific public (via social media and internet):

    - Abuse: Some members of the public do not like answers that they do not want to hear and can get abusive.
    - Legal aspects: Advice/opinions given over limited information and presented this way should be taken in the context of clinical pictures. It should be made clear that this is an opinion, and a clinical judgment should be made by the treating doctor. Advice on treatment (drugs) should be avoided over internet/social media, as other medical history information needs to be taken in consideration. Wrong interpretation/understanding can lead to legal ramifications.

7. Summary and the Future

Given the decreasing expertise in medical parasitology, this type of diagnostic help will become common and convenient. A team of experts can be put together from various parts of the world, and images and questions can be shared over electronic media. Additionally, sending bits of specimens by post to experts anywhere in the world is now possible in case molecular techniques are required for diagnosis. However, the legal aspects of giving advice and possible abuse over electronic or social media should be kept in mind.

Conflicts of Interest: The author declares no conflict of interest.

References

1. Crowe, A.; Koehler, A.V.; Sheorey, H.; Tolpinrud, A.; Gasser, R.B. PCR-coupled sequencing achieves specific diagnosis of onchocerciasis in a challenging clinical case, to underpin effective treatment and clinical management. *Infect. Genet. Evol.* **2018**, *66*, 192–194. [CrossRef] [PubMed]
2. Lim, C.K.; Crawford, A.; Moore, C.V.; Gasser, R.B.; Nelson, R.; Koehler, A.V.; Bradbury, R.S.; Speare, R.; Dhatrak, D.; Weldhagen, G.F. First human case of fatal Halicephalobus gingivalis meningoencephalitis in Australia. *J. Clin. Microbiol.* **2015**, *53*, 1768–1774. [CrossRef] [PubMed]
3. McKelvie, P.; Reardon, K.; Bond, K.; Spratt, D.M.; Gangell, A.; Zochling, J.; Daffy, J. A further patient with parasitic myositis due to Haycocknema perplexum, a rare entity. *J. Clin. Neurosci.* **2013**, *20*, 1019–1022. [CrossRef] [PubMed]
4. Koehler, A.V.; Spratt, D.M.; Norton, R.; Warren, S.; Mcewan, B.; Urkude, R.; Murth, S.; Robertson, T.; Mccallum, N.; Parsonson, F.; et al. More parasitic myositis cases in humans in Australia, and the definition of genetic markers for the causative agents as a basis for molecular diagnosis. *Infect. Genet. Evol.* **2016**, *44*, 69–75. [CrossRef] [PubMed]

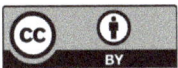

© 2020 by the author. Licensee MDPI, Basel, Switzerland. This article is an open access article distributed under the terms and conditions of the Creative Commons Attribution (CC BY) license (http://creativecommons.org/licenses/by/4.0/).

MDPI
St. Alban-Anlage 66
4052 Basel
Switzerland
Tel. +41 61 683 77 34
Fax +41 61 302 89 18
www.mdpi.com

Tropical Medicine and Infectious Disease Editorial Office
E-mail: tropicalmed@mdpi.com
www.mdpi.com/journal/tropicalmed

www.ingramcontent.com/pod-product-compliance
Lightning Source LLC
LaVergne TN
LVHW070543100526
838202LV00012B/359